Conversations in A
From insight to good practice

Paula Johnston and Sue Hatton

British Library Cataloguing in Publication Data

A CIP record for this book is available from the Public Library

ISBN 1 904082 69 6

© Copyright 2003 BILD Publications

BILD Publications is the publishing office of the
British Institute of Learning Disabilities
Campion House
Green Street
Kidderminster
Worcs
DY10 1JL
Telephone: 01562 723010
Fax: 01562 723029
e-mail: enquiries@bild.org.uk
Website: www.bild.org.uk

Please contact BILD for a free publications catalogue listing BILD
books, reports and training materials.

BILD Publications are distributed worldwide by
Plymbridge Distributors Limited
Plymbridge House
Estover Road
Plymouth
United Kingdom
PL6 7PZ
Telephone: 01752 202301
Fax: 01752 202333

Dedication

Paula:

"I would like to dedicate this book to all autistic people everywhere."

Sue:

"I would like to dedicate this book to the children at Coddington Court School and the staff who seek a better understanding of their autism in order to work more effectively with them. May this help a little."

Contents

Foreword

Over recent years, several biographies have been written by individuals with autistic spectrum disorders. These provide extremely useful insights into how they perceive and experience the world. For many years prior to this, those without autistic spectrum disorders (neurotypical people) speculated on autism and only a partial picture was obtained. This book brings the two perspectives together, based on conversations between the two authors. Paula Johnston, a woman with Asperger syndrome, presents events from her life and Sue Hatton, an experienced teacher, comments on the different interpretations that each has on the same scenario and points out the implications for those working and living with individuals with an asd.

People with an asd themselves, and those who work in this field, suggest that individuals with an asd should be viewed as different, rather than disordered or deficient, and that their view of the world and their wishes should be respected and valued. Neurotypical people need to consult and collaborate with them in reaching solutions rather than imposing strategies and interventions which they deem to be in the best interests of the person.

Paula's interpretations of events and her responses to situations will not be shared by all people with an asd, but, as Sue points out, from her teaching experience, many children have acted in similar ways to particular situations. Common messages from these and other adult biographies emerge which have significant implications for practice. Specifically, the need to have time and space to be alone; the stress of social situations; their response to being touched; their difficulties in carrying out everyday tasks, despite high intellectual ability; the role of special interests and the length of time needed to process information.

In Paula's accounts, the failure of neurotypical people to understand her perspective and response is clear. When asked what is most difficult about their lives, individuals with an asd often say '*other people*'. When asked what would be most helpful, some say, people who do not make assumptions about our needs and who try to understand us. This book vividly portrays the intense reactions and feelings that Paula experiences in relation to everyday events. It is exhausting to read at times, and her levels of anxiety are palpable. These accounts help us, as neurotypicals, to understand behaviours which seem odd and extreme, but which to the person with an asd are normal and logical. The commentary provided by Sue Hatton on Paula's explanations and the neurotypical position provides teaching staff and parents with much to consider when making appropriate responses and creating effective interventions to support individuals with an asd. This book then is a very welcome addition to the literature written by those people with an asd.

Glenys Jones
Lecturer in autism
University of Birmingham
May 2003

The Introduction

Asperger syndrome is such a hidden disability. We are so good at learning, imitating and covering up, but sometimes covering up is just not enough.

I always find my own peer group the most difficult to be accepted by. One day (when I was much younger) I decided to try. I got some of the kind of clothes they wore, the high heel shoes, etc from a charity shop and fixed my hair like they had it at the time. As I was gazing into a shop window a woman of my age group, and similarly attired, got out of a car and approached the shop. She turned to me (just before entering the shop) and smiled saying, "Can you watch my car?" "Yes," I replied, without understanding. I looked at the car, it was boring and I couldn't see what purpose that would serve. So I started to look again in the shop window. Then I heard a noise behind me. I looked round and saw a traffic warden stick a piece of paper on her car. I realised I was somehow supposed to have prevented this happening, but I didn't know how. Then I saw the woman coming towards the door of the shop, and, dreading meeting her, I ran off very fast. That's the last time I tried to copy members of my peer group.

Paula Johnston

For those of you who have read even one other book about someone with Asperger syndrome or by someone with an autistic spectrum disorder (asd) this may appear as just another funny anecdote about the literal interpretation people with an asd tend to take on language. For others this may be a revelation and the one story you remember and re-tell when you have the opportunity to try and explain the nature of asd to someone else. There is no doubt that listening to people who have Asperger syndrome or reading their books is one of the best ways to learn what it is like. If we can do this, we are so much better equipped to work with children, young people, adults with an asd and their families who do not have this insight. It enables us to be so much more effective if we recognise the very different way of functioning that children, young people and adults with an asd have, in our play groups, schools, colleges and the workplace.

My hope for this book is that it will do more than I have described, important though that is. For me, the insights and experiences that Paula is able and happy to share about her life help to unlock some of the mystery that surrounds children, young people and adults with an asd who do not speak or write about their lives and are also labelled as having a severe learning disability.

I now find myself back where I began my working life in a specialist school for children with an asd (though in 1973 it was not an educational establishment but a hospital, and the children were on a ward and not in a classroom). I also run training events, often with the help of Paula. As we travel home from different places, I have shared with Paula the confusing behaviour of many of the children who live in this residential special school and so often she sheds light and suggests something I, or any of the staff, have not considered. We are struggling to think autistically in order to get alongside these children and find ways of working with them that will enable them to be fully included members of our society. For Paula, thinking autistically comes quite naturally and so the idea of this book and of us writing it together was formed.

At the various training events and conferences where Paula has spoken, people often ask, "Why don't you write a book, what you are sharing is so helpful?" What I keep seeing is just how valuable Paula's insights into her own life experience are for those with an asd who do not speak and are not able to communicate their experience of the world to us in a way that we understand – and so we all struggle.

With Paula's help I hope the struggle for some can be made a little less arduous.

Sue Hatton

Chapter 1

How people see me – disruptive or retarded

As a child I have been accused of attention seeking and disruptive behaviour. If I could have read the situation, or understood other people's ideas or expectations, my life would have been different. To ascribe the more usual motives to an Asperger syndrome person's inappropriate behaviour won't be fitting.

In home economics class, despite 'A' grade essays in nutrition, I would repeatedly overflow the sink or put on the gas without lighting the cooker. Having seen my written work the teachers assumed that this behaviour was deliberately meant to cause trouble. I was labelled disruptive and accused of attention seeking. That is unlikely, as to be disruptive you need to know what is going on around you, to understand what other people's expectations are and what upsets them. The child with an autistic spectrum disorder will be misreading the situation.

Sue comments: Paula puts this in such a matter of fact way that there is a danger we read it and don't take in the reality of what she is saying and begin to apply it. Some of the most frequent comments I hear about a child is that he or she is attention seeking, deliberately awkward, rude, cheeky, disruptive, etc. This may be said of a child with a diagnosis of Asperger syndrome who is in a mainstream educational setting, or it may be a child with a diagnosis of autism and learning difficulties in a very specialist educational setting. Wherever the situation, we need to think long and hard about what Paula is telling us. With no real awareness or understanding of what the people around her expect, or what might upset them or wind them up, she is not capable of consciously behaving in any of the ways that have been described.

My experience with staff in schools and many other settings and also my personal experience is that we may think we know and understand but time and time again we show that we don't.

The child with autism who keeps putting things down the toilet is seen as mischievous and then devious as the child appears to wait until your back is turned in order to be able to do the deed.

The child with autism who is said to be a constant tease or bully with other children in the class because he or she pinches and pokes them or calls them names.

I could go on giving example after example of behaviour that gets wrongly ascribed and therefore the individual who gets wrongly labelled. It seems so difficult for us to stop making these assumptions that Paula talks of and to learn to think in a more autistic way – to put on our 'Asperger lens' (Cumine, Leach and Stevenson, 1998).

One Saturday night I was at a barn dance or square dance. When the instructions were given I thought I understood them. I felt OK as we stood in our groups of four, but when we all lined up to face each other I was no longer sure who was in my group and who wasn't. When the music started I could see lots of people dashing off in directions that I couldn't predict. While attempting the back-to-back with my partner, on trying to return to my original place, I had several collisions with other dancers and ousted several ladies from their positions by ending up opposite their partner. I gatecrashed several groups as they danced in circles, being unable to find my own group. In other words, I managed single-handedly to cause general chaos. Afterwards people said very kindly words to this effect, "Well done dear, you did very well." They treated me like I was retarded.

Sue comments: The difficulties that Paula has with co-ordination and recognition of faces all seem to relate to her sensory processing and we know that for people with an asd "their sensory perception and responses may be different." (Jones, 2002). However, their differences are not all similar. This makes it difficult in relation to understanding how the senses work with various people with an asd. It also means that again we often make mistakes in the assumptions we make and therefore the strategies we may try to put in place to be supportive or teach a child with an asd.

For many people reading the description that Paula shares of being clumsy, having poor coordination and being confused by people's faces, may be far removed from the experience of another individual with an asd who is very agile, can climb fences and balance on high walls with no fear.

Exactly how the senses are different for the individual with an asd can be extremely varied and that is what we need to remember most. As we seek to be alongside and understand the individual and their triad of impairment (difficulties with communication, social interaction and inflexibility of thought) and their individual way of sensing the world, we will begin to help them write their own manual for the best ways of working with them. It is very individual and so often goes against the natural ways many of us think and our usually helpful intuition. To accept this we have to dig deep into our set ways of thinking and change.

I sometimes have difficulty understanding verbal instructions. As I am no longer trying to get and hold down a job this shows itself mainly when I am out shopping.

Recently I went for a coffee in a shopping centre at one of those counters. There were two girls facing me from behind the counter. The one to my right asked me what I would like. I pointed out the cake I wanted, which she fetched. She laid the tray for me and made the coffee. When asked how much it was she told me the price. I tried to hand her the money, she didn't take it and said, "Give the money to Angela" (or some similar name). I heard the words, English is my first language, but somehow the meaning didn't register with me. She continued to repeat the phrase, while I wondered why she wouldn't take the money. It was only at the third time of hearing it, but still with no real understanding, that I realised the other girl behind the counter, to my left, was stood behind the cash register. She had her hand outstretched, as I belatedly realised, probably to receive my money. So I put the money in her hand and things began to go normally again.

In these instances it is as if time stands still. The very ordinary words reach me, but somehow there is a time delay between my hearing them and my understanding the meaning and thus being able to act on it. The social interaction stops. I stop what I am doing. The other person stops what they are doing as they repeat the words. Then, after what seems to me like a long time span my bewilderment wears off and I understand, act appropriately and the other person reacts to this and things proceed normally.

Once, I was standing in a queue in Sainsbury's, directly behind a young woman whose purchases had just been checked through and she was giving the checkout girl her money. Suddenly she turned towards me and said, "Would you have two pence?" I heard the words but couldn't understand. She repeated the phrase, as I stood confused. Then the woman immediately behind me in the queue pushed past me and put something into the hand of the girl. "Here's two pence love," she said. Then the girl gave the money to the checkout girl who said, "You've got a £2.50 voucher, would you like to leave it or take it?" "I'll take it," the girl said. Then she pushed past me and gave it to the woman behind me, saying, "Please have this and thanks for helping me out of an embarrassing situation." She glowered at me as she left. By this time I had assessed the situation and was quite disappointed about missing out on earning a £2.50 voucher.

Sue comments: This is another really helpful story from Paula to remind us of the problems with communication and the length of time it can take someone with an asd to process language directed at them and in particular when the words are not expected.

I find myself talking about this aspect of the triad of impairments very regularly when talking to groups of parents and professionals in a wide range of settings. It is something I know about. It is a problem I am quick to spot when observing in a classroom setting or a residential home for adults. However, when I am teaching on a Monday afternoon and one of the teenagers with autism looks at me strangely, I find myself repeating a phrase or rewording it. I find it so hard to just wait and allow the processing to happen in that longer time span that Paula describes so vividly. If I can make the conscious effort to speak and then let time stand still for a few extra seconds – it works! Understanding comes and I get an answer or an appropriate response. But it is so hard to do, especially for teachers like myself who have spent years finding new ways to explain things. Teachers, and others, are prepared to elaborate, repeat and give added and additional explanation because we care and we want the learning to take place. But with the individual with an asd what we really need to do is be quiet once the first simple explanation has been given containing key words. **We need to wait . . .**

Having said all that, perhaps one of the most revealing things about Paula's experience in that supermarket queue is how she explains what she felt when she understood what was said and what was occurring socially. Paula comprehended both the words and the actions eventually. Was she then embarrassed or anxious about having made a social gaff? No – that is how I would have felt and as I read the account it was what I was expecting because that would be the natural reaction for me and many other people. But to expect that from Paula is again not thinking autistically. Paula does not feel embarrassed, she does not have any sense of a social gaff, but she would have liked the £2.50 voucher! Does that then make her self-centred? No, she has Asperger syndrome and her confused reactions to both the language spoken and then to the social setting are due to that fact. The Asperger syndrome doesn't disappear with that additional timespan required to process the spoken language. So, for Paula, the key factor in that story was the concrete £2.50 voucher and not the range of feelings being expressed by everyone else involved in that scenario. How easy to wrongly label her, even with a certain level of understanding.

A common occurrence is when I go to a checkout and the girl repeats two or three times, "I'm closed, love", before I understand and go to another checkout. No one in these situations has ever said the word retarded to me but on occasions I have been asked if I am deaf.

The first time I actually heard myself referred to as retarded was in the first office I worked in, having arrived in London back from India. I was about 22 years old. A woman working with me told the boss quite openly in my presence, "She's a bit retarded." I was surprised because all the failures and rejections I was to suffer were still ahead of me. But it was in some way a kind of release. I had been struggling so hard to cover up difficulties in that job. Later in nursing, when a fellow student said to me, "Paula you're disorientated", that was something I could heartily agree with!

Chapter 2

Social interaction – my likes and dislikes

Social interactions I don't like

I don't like having to make the effort to chat and not being able to think about what I want to think about. I don't like having to fit into other people's scenarios. If they talk about characters in soaps, for instance, I don't know what they mean. I never watch them. I had to endure some of that while looking after my mother. I used to try to stand it, counting the moments. Sometimes I had to get out before I had made her cup of tea or whatever, as I couldn't endure any more of her words in my mind.

If people express opinions about something real, for instance something that has been on the news, if my opinion is opposite I will say so, and explain why I hold my view even if their reaction is hostile. It really hurts me to have someone else's opinion on something important squashing mine. I feel so sure and so right about what I think.

I don't feel any need for social interaction. Left to my own devices, I am never bored or lonely. I only get bored if, for instance, I am waiting in the doctor's surgery and there is music playing. I can't put my earphones in (with something of interest to me which I have recorded, *in my own voice)* as I might miss my turn.

Social interaction is nonsensical. The neighbour I had tried to be friendly with once brought a bird to keep in a cage, she said the bird was supposed to sing. It is only the males of that species that sing and so far it had not sung at all. I said that perhaps it was a female and she told me that the man who had sold it to her knew that it was a male because he had swung a stone on some string in front of the bird! The man had told her that if it swung from side to side it was a male bird and if it was female it would rotate. I asked how and she told me it was to do with the vibrations! I asked her if it was the string that vibrated and how could that possibly happen? She replied, telling me that the bird made it happen. So I said, "There is nothing about a bird which can make an object vibrate." "It's scientific," she said. I said, "If that was the case, whether a bird is male or female, when broken down it is composed of the same substances and would affect the swinging stone in the same way. You need to take the bird to a proper pet shop or to the animal hospital and have it examined." She became angry and dashed off. To me, this was nonsensical and not scientific.

Social interaction is boring. It may be about characters in films or soaps. I have no interest to hear about these people who do not exist and about events that have never happened. They claim that these soaps deal with social problems but there are plenty of documentaries dealing with the real lives of real people. Social interaction is to pass the time for them, not for my benefit.

Once, I was in the waiting room of the hospital, waiting while my husband was having chemotherapy. I had my earphones in. I became aware that a lady was trying to speak to me; I removed my earphones and gave her my attention. She asked the time. I looked at my watch, told her the time and then replaced my earphones. I saw her looking around and then begin to speak to another lady. I removed my earphones in time to hear the lady tell her the time. Soon the two of them were engaged in an animated conversation. I thought she was just trying to use me to pass the time for her.

One of the problems at work was the social side; everyone talked about soaps or films, which I absolutely hate. All about families and relationships, which don't interest me at all. I haven't much experience of work; my special interests have led me to voluntary work, where of course the conversation is more interesting and relevant for me. During work I tended to sit and think inside myself about my interests while others chatted on. I didn't join in until suddenly someone mentioned something of interest to me, then I would launch into a lengthy animated discourse, leaving the others quite surprised, with remarks like, "I didn't know you had a tongue in your head, love," or words to that effect. Then I would again lapse into silent reflection on my own preoccupations. Other people seem to go to work for social reasons while I would go to perform a specific task, but that is not enough. They also want you to pass their time for them as though they do not know what to do.

One of the benefits of a diagnosis is the relief, losing the feeling of guilt at not achieving in terms of career and relationships. I am married to a man 18 years older than me with asd traits – he saves egg cartons, yoghurt cartons, empty washing powder boxes, etc and becomes distressed at attempts to remove them. We have no children as we found normal physical relations difficult. He was a special interest of mine for about nine months, during which time we got married. Unfortunately he is no longer a special interest. I desperately need to be alone a lot of each day. I consider my time spent in company as 'being in public' and after a few hours if the other person doesn't go away I will run out. That's the only way of staving off a tantrum when I will scream and cry loudly for hours. So I need to get out and if I meet someone who knows me I can't afford to acknowledge them. I have to get away. I get frustrated with my husband's loud TV and radio programmes. I have hit him and banged my head against the wall, etc. Things are much better since we have had separate rooms. I find the whole relationship difficult but I have been homeless three times and I need a roof over my head.

A relationship is very difficult and very frustrating but if an autistic person can endure it, it has great benefits in developing social skills. You are forced to endure eye contact, physical contact, to negotiate what is going to happen during the day. That's the most frustrating thing. When my husband is away I happily get up and go out where I want, when I want, which is natural for me to do even when he is there. But I find I have to compromise and fit in, to some extent, with him. It's not natural for me to compromise, but if you can learn to, it's of great benefit for interacting with people in society.

I did briefly have a female friend. I took interest in everything she was interested in and, for instance, bought her purple jewellery or whatever, as she was fond of purple. I also researched which foods had less than 4% fat for her as she frequently tried to diet. But I had to give it up. We went on a day trip, which I found beyond endurance. I thought if I was on my own I could read with my coffee and I could listen to a tape I had recorded about something I want to learn rather than listen to all this talking. It was with great difficulty that I managed not to scream with frustration or run away. On other occasions, when out for too long in company I have just disappeared without explanation, which is preferable to having a tantrum that is difficult to stop once it has started.

The woman I tried to be friends with would sometimes come in when my husband went out to a music event or something. I had waited so long for him to go out so I could work on something I was interested in without interruption or having to wear earplugs. So if she came I found it difficult not to let my upset show. I began not answering the door. She understood and put a note through the letterbox, "I hope you are enjoying your free time," a phrase I use a lot. I realised that like a lot of people I have met she was so desperate not to be alone that she would listen to me talk incessantly about my current interest. I thought, I don't have to do this, there must be someone equally desperate and the two of them can pass the time for each other. So I finished that and have not entered into another relationship of that nature.

Social interactions I do like
I am interested in understanding different religions. You cannot really understand them just from books. You will end up knowing more about a specific religion as regards its scriptural content, etc than the ordinary practitioner does but without actually knowing a practitioner you will never know about their folk beliefs and practices. For that reason I enjoyed visiting and having round to my place once or twice a Muslim girl called Khalida. She washed her hands, etc and performed her prayers in my presence and she also told me in great detail what the Ayatollah Khomeini wore, the precepts he kept and how he was going to come from France to Iran to reform the country. It was exciting to see him on the TV. He looked so handsome and I knew so much about him, so I followed the progress of the country and it did indeed turn out very well.

I take great interest in people; I have a lot of love for them. I like to find out about their culture and to give money in an emergency. But it is all in the abstract. I would have been a lot less enthusiastic if Khalida had asked me to go up town shopping with her, I would probably have found it beyond endurance. It's the same with the Buddhist temple I attend. Before I actually went I read avidly about the kind of Buddhism. It is the Mahayana, original fundamentalist, very strict at keeping the rules. So I really learned all about that before I went to the temple. For instance, females cannot have physical contact with the monks. You cannot touch them or their robes or hand something directly to them. Also if talking to a monk, whether you are male or female, if the monk is sitting you should not stand above them, you should get down to their level even if there is no seat. It's the tradition, so I enjoyed this very much. I know what to do and how to do it. I can do it very successfully and having read so much about it I am able to be with the monks and interact with them. I find this thrilling and it brings it all to life.

There is a woman from another temple who comes to our temple for Buddhism class. I enjoy talking to her about Buddhism. She tells me what the monk said in her meditation class, about the Buddhist books she is reading or about the retreats she regularly attends. She does not talk to me about anything else at all. (I have explained to her about my syndrome and given her some literature about it so she is very understanding.) She and the other ladies who come to class often talk about other things such as their families, eg grandchildren or the films they have gone out to see. The others have tried to include me but I just drift off and wash the dishes or something. But Leila never ever talks to me about anything except Buddhism.

I also enjoy interacting with the people who have been born Buddhist, because unlike the books which deal with the sometimes mind-blowing doctrines, from them I can learn the folk beliefs and practices. They are happy to teach me and pleased that I am so keen to learn. The result of this again is that some people have wanted me to go shopping with them, etc and I have had to excuse myself or they would be shocked at the tantrum I may possibly have. I care a lot and have sponsored two orphan girls and made other donations but it has to be in the abstract.

The temple is two, or it can be three, bus journeys away from where I live and this is an important feature. Because there is someone else in the house where I live I feel stressful. So I need the two bus journeys on my own to relax and to be able to interact in the temple. If someone sat with me on the bus and spoke to me then by the time I got to the temple I would already have had as much social interaction as I can stand. That is why I say three buses sometimes – on the rare occasions someone I've met from somewhere, or for some other reason, sits beside me and starts to talk I will get off the bus and catch another one. I make sure I'm in a receptive state ready to communicate when I do get to the temple. I just want to go there to explore my own interest and learn. I am not looking for company or friendship, I don't want to know the people that I meet there more intimately or to meet them socially outside the temple.

One of the things I do at the temple is clean the toilets and I like the routine I have worked out for myself. One week my routine was disrupted and it put me off and upset me. Normally I just go, do my three toilets and leave. It's a very satisfying achievement. But one week my meditation teacher said two lots of toilets are enough, "Don't work so hard, relax and talk." When I'm there I answer the door to other people who come and talk about their problems, etc while I just do the work and then leave. Perhaps he thought I was feeling left out and he should give me some time. But I find talking much more stressful than toilet cleaning. Anyhow I told him I was giving a talk and I have this syndrome. He said, "Well, you work much better than someone who is not sick." It is true because other people who go there to work talk amongst themselves, which I try to avoid. They phone people and play music. So, although they can work much more easily and quickly than I can, I actually get much more done in the time because I am not social.

One advantage of this syndrome is that I am quite happy just to work on and on. I'm never bored or lonely. I never do something just to pass the time. This phrase other people use means nothing to me, and I never say, "Whatever will I do, there is nothing good on TV tonight," as I have heard other people say. I only watch TV when there is something I need to find out about. I always know what I want to do. The trouble is if someone or something stands in my way of doing what I want to do. This results in frustration, tantrums and even violence. But, left alone I can produce a lot of good work.

I'm having some difficulties with the temple at the moment. There is a girl who seems to live near me. I saw her at the bus stop. I thought

I should speak to her and she told me she had seen me at a special event at the temple. I thought it would be nice if she could help me with my Tibetan language and Tibetan cookery and I could help her with her English. That is all to do with my special interest, after all. But she is very 'normal'. She probably loves films, soaps, pop music and I'm not normal. Frank, my husband, isn't 'normal'. The house is like a tip with all the paper and second hand clothes, etc. If I was living alone I could probably manage about once a week to see someone. But I am already at screaming point with Frank. I just can't take on anyone else. So I gave her my phone number, but not my address. Next time I saw her she did not return my smile, she looked very unfriendly. I felt unable to attend the last special event as she would be there as well as some other people who want to be more friendly.

When I lived with my mother and was looking after her, quite frequently she had to go into hospital for a few days. I used to visit her in the evening and then look forward to going home to the flat, free from the TV, free from her calling me, but inevitably someone from her flat complex would see me arrive and soon after I got back the door would knock and I would have to endure hours of talking. So I began sneaking round the back way, then I wouldn't put the lights on. The toilet and bathroom had no window. I could put the light on in there but it activated the fan which made it a bit cool, but I put on the heater. I would make myself a drink in the dark and take my books into the bathroom from about 8pm to 12:30am – pure pleasure. But even that didn't work, someone saw me making a drink in the dark and came ringing the doorbell. So I stopped coming back. I visited my mum with all my books, writing material and tape machine in my bag on my back. Tuesdays and Thursdays I could stay in the reference library till 9pm. Other evenings I stayed in one of the many hospital waiting areas on another floor with the coffee machine, toilet and lots of space. If someone came along and started to talk I would just take the lift to a more or less identical waiting area on another floor.

I had the same trouble where I live now when I was friendly with the neighbours. On Sunday while Frank was at the Quaker meeting, I enjoyed using the kitchen area to do some reading, etc. But in the good weather the neighbour and her boyfriend would do some gardening. They could see right into my kitchen. I had agreed to see her twice a week already, but it wasn't enough. If they saw me they would come in for coffee. So instead of using the kitchen table I had to sit on the floor to do my work. I had to crawl on my hands and knees to switch on the kettle which was fortunately out of sight and also crawl to the toilet.

While nurse training I found the strain of working and living in the hospital too much and I point blank refused to go out with anyone from the hospital when I was off duty. I really needed to get away from everything to do with the hospital. But one day another student from my group insisted on following me. I really needed to get away on my own, but she wouldn't take no for an answer. I tried to be friendly on the bus, we got to the town, but after about one hour I could not take anymore. I vanished without explanation. She was from overseas. She didn't speak much English. How she got back to the hospital, I don't know, I didn't ask and she didn't speak to me again anyway. I had no intention of leaving her stranded. I didn't think about that. I just felt I was losing control and might do something drastic. So it was better to get away. I have felt the same way often, eg, when I was with my husband and we missed a connection between trains travelling back from Dublin. I was OK about it and thought I could just have a coffee and look at one of my books. But my husband continued to talk about missing the connection. I said "OK, it happened, it's over now, don't prolong it by talking about it." But he continued to talk about it. So I swung my rucksack and hit him with it, then ran off shouting, "I'll be back in twenty minutes before the next train, don't follow me and then I can calm down." I dived into a coffee shop on my own. I had felt the same way with that student nurse. I was on the point of raising my carrier bag with two jars of Marks & Spencer jam to thump her when instead I dived into a store and out the back entrance. People just don't understand!

Sue comments: I have only known Paula about eighteen months but there are times when I speak about her and I have found myself referring to Paula as, 'my friend!' It is, of course, so natural for me to do this. I enjoy getting to know new people and making new friends in different areas of my life. I enjoy talking about relationships and being a part of many friendship circles. This makes listening to some of what Paula has to share on this topic difficult. I feel I want her to experience life differently – I also feel at times that people make a whole range of wrong assumptions about Paula that would not happen if they knew her a little better.

Paula does refer to her husband, Frank, as a special interest from the past and who she now finds it hard to live with as he gets in the way of her plans for the day. However, Paula is an excellent carer and Frank needs daily physical care since he had his operation for cancer. Paula fulfils this role with thought and exactness. She wants and needs her own space and she is quick to let you know that, but she also shows her ability to take care of someone and to fit her life around the needs of someone who requires Paula's support to live and function each day.

I also have no doubt that Paula takes enjoyment in the planned meetings we have to write this book, and to prepare for some training we are doing together. The important thing is for me to see Paula's need to know exactly why I am coming, what is expected from her and when I will leave. There is a lack of spontaneity in the friendship but there is a security in the dependability of Paula to do what she has said she will do. There is also opportunity for laughter as the two very different cultures that we exist in meet.

On one occasion when driving back from some training, Paula turned to me and said, "What are you doing this weekend, Sue?" Surprised by this request to know something about me, I was silent for a moment and then asked her if she really wanted to know, as that was an unusual question for her to ask me. Her reply came swiftly – "Well, no Sue, I don't really want to know, but it is the sort of thing people ask isn't it and I was just hoping that your answer wouldn't be too long or too boring!"

I said that we did not need to talk and so we drove the hour journey home in what I would call a companiable silence, Paula lost in her own thoughts and me wondering what they might be about!

People who work with children who have a diagnosis of autism often ask me about how much they should do to bring them out of 'their' world and to encourage interaction with people in 'our' world. My response is to say a bit of both. It is about respecting the need to be left alone, to take on board what we hear able people with an asd telling us. However, we also have a duty to encourage and teach the value of social interaction to a certain extent and not let the problems it may cause mean we leave the child in the corner of the room all the time lost in their own world. I don't think it is about finding the 'real' child or person within the autistic personality. I think it is about respect for difference and support for living in a society that thrives on social interaction.

I suggested to Paula and her husband that they might find value in having a circle of friends set up − a small group of people who they know and who can help where help is needed, and who would meet with them on a regular basis. Frank was a little reluctant but Paula has soon grasped the value of such a group of people. She sees it as an opportunity to get things done, with help and to learn new skills. (Recently this has included learning to empty the vacuum cleaner and use the cash point machine.)

Both Frank and Paula like the planning and predictability that goes with this type of organised social interaction. There is a mutual benefit to these social times for me as well. Getting to know Paula better and gaining insight into the nature of her asd continues to help my work with children who have an additional learning disability.

Circles of friends are most commonly used in schools to help a range of children with special educational needs cope socially in the school environment. However, I believe there is much greater scope to be had from this concept for adults with an autistic spectrum disorder (Hatton, 2002).

Chapter 3

Why my opinion is right!

Taking sides

In secondary school I was completely isolated. I didn't share values, beliefs, likes and dislikes with anyone else. I hadn't been socialised, as everyone else seemed to have been. Probably in those early years, when others reputedly imbibe the values of the group they belong to, I hadn't been aware of what was going on. Now, as a teenager I was quite aware but the subtleties of the Northern Irish divided society escaped me. I was dimly aware that I was expected to be on some side or other. But I didn't see why I should be. I considered this to be an imposition, a restriction of my liberty. I was perfectly confident about my views. I felt I was right (I still do) and I was ready to point out where others were wrong (I don't do that quite so much any more). I didn't share their culture. I was a stranger and treated as such.

Why I am right

The side one is on is not hereditary. It is not genetically passed on like the colour of one's eyes. There is therefore absolutely no reason to accept and perpetuate the ethos of one's family group, etc. Rather, one should examine the evidence of the relative merit of one's family's position and the opposing one and make an informed choice. For example, the Protestant side is good because it has the tradition to dress smartly and not to drink alcohol. On the other hand the Catholic side has the monastic tradition, which is also good. A better choice is Mahayana Buddhism, which incorporates both these advantages having both the tradition to dress up smartly and to avoid alcohol and also having the monastic tradition.

Sue comments: I found this explanation of why Paula has chosen Buddhism amusing – though of course Paula does not see it like that and thinks I am wrong. To me, Paula has taken things that she thinks are a part of a particular religion/denomination that I don't think are necessarily true anyway. She then puts them together to fit what she likes in a certain form of Buddhism. It seems just daft to me – but to her it is real and logical.

Let us think of an adult with learning difficulties and autism who collects boxes and packaging and whose room is piled high with months of collecting. To me, it seems daft! Why aren't they keen to collect something more interesting? What is the point of having piles of boxes in your room which once placed there you do nothing with? Then, if someone tries to move them or get rid of them, major anxiety is caused and no explanation will suffice, even if understood. But the boxes help the person with an asd. They enable the person to feel they have some control over life in a very confusing world. They may cope better with confusion and change outside their own room as long as the boxes within their room remain secure and the same.

With better understanding we may learn to leave the issue of the boxes but too often that is not the case.

The opticians

When I was about nine years old my mother took me with her when she accompanied her friend, who wore glasses, along to the opticians for a check up. After she was finished the optician asked my mother to have a check up. She said she didn't have any problems with her eyesight and that she was just there with a friend. But the optician persuaded her and she came out with a prescription for both distance and reading glasses. Then he asked me to come in to have my sight tested. I refused. I ran out of the shop but not before telling the optician, "This is just a trick. If anyone comes in here you will tell them that they need glasses. Well, you're not going to do that to me." The truth was, I had quite a lot of difficulty seeing things far away. But I didn't see why that should be a problem. Far away things ought to be less clear. If you want to see them in more detail you can just walk closer to them. Anyway I wasn't going to give in. So every year, when the medical people came to my school, as I stood in the queue, I memorised each line of the eye test card which was on the wall beside us, so when it came to my turn I could read it perfectly to the bottom line, and I was never prescribed glasses!

Why I am right

Firstly, an optician's is not a charity. It is a business with a quota to fulfil. Therefore an optician will sell you as many pairs of spectacles as they can, whether you need them or not. Secondly, we should remember that sight is not simply a matter of light impinging on the eyes. It is also a matter of interpretation by the brain (of the corresponding signals which reach the visual area of the brain). This interpretation is partly based on previous experiences. Therefore, by familiarising ourselves with our environment we can learn to match what we see with what is actually there. Anyhow, no human being or animal can really see what is actually 'out there'. What we see is limited and filtered by the particular type of eye we have whether human or animal. So why should you present your brain with another set of incomplete information to interpret, that is different to what you have already available without glasses? Anyhow, glasses cause dependency. They have to be replaced at least every two years, and if lost or broken the brain will have great difficulty interpreting the signals that come to it via the eye, until the glasses are replaced. This is partly because after a period of wearing glasses, you will see less clearly, as I certainly did after being forced to wear glasses on the ward during my two attempts at nurse training. I am right because other people's prescriptions change and they seem to need increasingly stronger glasses, while my prescription stays the same, probably partly because I remember the letters of the testing chart.

Nurse training

One week while nurse training it was my duty to serve the food to patients in their own private rooms. I went to the kitchen as instructed. The meals with metal covers were all put on the trolley and I delivered them, according to room number, starting with the room next to the kitchen and working my way down to the furthest room. As the week went on the patients in the first few rooms closest to the kitchen thanked me and said "It is wonderful having you bringing the meals. At last we are getting our food hot." I thought I must be delivering it faster than the other nurses. Then by about day four, just as I was leaving the kitchen with the trolley, the ward sister appeared and shouted, "Nurse, everybody else always wheels the trolley down to the end of the corridor and serves the food to the room furthest from the kitchen and works her way back to the room beside the kitchen. But you have to do it the opposite way to everybody else; you have to do it your own way. Well, I won't have it."

I was amazed at this outburst. Firstly, I just had never noticed that the other nurses served the food the opposite way to how I did it. Secondly, had I noticed that I would not have considered it a valid reason for me to alter my habit of doing the task in what I considered to be the best way. Anyway the extra journey entailed in their method must make everyone's meal on average colder. I can't remember my exact reaction to her outburst but one thing is for sure, somebody else had to serve the food. This kind of thing has happened so many times in work, when I have for some time performed a task so perfectly and carefully, put so much effort into a routine, then someone will come and demand that I do it in a different way. I just can't do it.

Why I am right – my method
Estimated time for food leaving oven to trolley, to kitchen exit = 30 seconds. Estimated time for moving from kitchen to room one or from room one to room two etc, each 30 seconds. Estimated time for serving food to patient = 30 seconds.

Patient (1) receives food after ½ + ½ + ½ = 1½ mins
Patient (2) receives food after 1½ + ½ + ½ = 2½ mins
Patient (3) receives food after 2½ + ½ + ½ = 3½ mins
Patient (4) receives food after 3½ + ½ + ½ = 4½ mins
Patient (5) receives food after 4½ + ½ + ½ = 5½ mins
Patient (6) receives food after 5½ + ½ + ½ = 6½ mins
Patient (7) receives food after 6½ + ½ + ½ = 7½ mins
Patient (8) receives food after 7½ + ½ + ½ = 8 ½ mins

Total 40 mins

Mean average of time patient receives food – 40 ÷ 8 = 5.
Mean average = 5 mins

Their method
Estimated time for food leaving oven to trolley to kitchen exit = 30 secs. Estimated time for moving from kitchen to room (8) = 4 mins

Patient (8) receives food after (4 + ½) = 4½ mins
Patient (7) receives food after (4½ + ½ + ½ = 5½ mins
Patient (6) receives food after (5½ + ½ + ½) = 6½ mins
Patient (5) receives food after (6½ + ½ + ½) = 7½ mins
Patient (4) receives food after (7½ + ½ + ½) = 8½ mins
Patient (3) receives food after (8½ + ½ + ½) = 9½ mins
Patient (2) receives food after (9½ + ½ + ½) = 10½ mins
Patient (1) receives food after (10½ + ½ + ½) = 11½ mins
Total = 64 mins

Mean average of time patient receives food 64 ÷ 8 = 8 minutes. Mean average = 8mins.

Mean difference between my method and their method = 8–5 = 3 mins. Therefore, by their method, on average patients receive their food three minutes later than by my method. Therefore my method is better and I am right.

PVS patient
One evening I was working alone with the Ward Sister. I had been studying about PVS patients, those people described as being in a permanent vegetative state. From the procedure book one of the facts I had memorised was that a PVS patient was not to be turned directly after a feed as the swallow mechanism doesn't function properly in someone who is unconscious and the patient may choke to death. As we had a patient on the ward with that condition, the Ward Sister agreed to show me how to prepare and administer a nasal-gastric feed. After that was completed the Sister asked me to help her turn the patient on to her other side. Remembering what I had just studied I said, "But it says in the procedure book that you must not turn a PVS patient after feeding, as there is a danger of them choking to death." "Oh, no, she will be just fine," the Sister tried to reassure me. But I repeated, "It says in the procedure book, etc, etc." "Look, I am in charge of this ward, and I'll decide if and when a patient should be turned." However I stuck to my position. "It says in the procedure book, etc."

The Sister accused me of trying to run her ward. Of course nothing could be further from the truth. It was just that I found the textbook information safe and dependable, tried and tested, giving control over the situation and offering a predictable outcome. To step outside that would be taking a frightening step into the unknown. And I just was not able to do that.

Why I am right
The patient fitted into the category of a PVS patient, she had just been fed. According to the procedures book, patients in this situation, if turned, are in danger of choking to death. These are the facts. There can be no argument about this. Feed + immediate turning = possible choking to death. For me to be willing to participate in turning the patient something in the equation would have to change. The patient would have to be re-classified as a non-PVS patient. This is not possible. The procedure book would have to be changed. This may be possible. Exceptions to the rule could be described together with verifiable evidence which could be checked. It would not be right to accept the Sister's judgement if it disagrees with the book because:

- the Sister may be fed up with the patient and want her to die
- she may not care whether the patient lives or dies, but want to get me into trouble
- she may just be stupid and unable to foresee the consequences of taking this course of action.

Where I am able to assess the situation, examine the facts and come to the correct decision, I can't easily relinquish this position.

Sue comments: How easily I can take the side of the Ward Sister – a busy woman running a busy ward. She knows her patients and is able to weigh up the pros and cons of different situations quite quickly. The procedure book was learnt and then adapted as her experience adapted the theories she knew. Then this young nurse not only questions her but continues to argue and make her statement about the 'procedure book'. To the Sister she has an arrogant 'know it all' on her hands – but that was also not true. The Sister had a keen and interested young student nurse with Asperger syndrome, who finds it almost impossible to imagine that anyone can think differently from herself, let alone go against a rule set out in a book.

We just don't realise how often, as adults, we change the rules, don't say what we mean, alter the plans, cope with an unplanned-for eventuality and this we do intuitively, quite naturally.

For Paula this makes the world non-sensical and frightening. Arguing does nothing to calm her fear or to bring order to the chaos that she sees surrounding the behaviour of that Ward Sister. She is not able to cope with an alteration in the procedure – even if the Sister had given her a reason there would still have been a major difficulty.

Let us think for a moment about the person with an autistic spectrum disorder who is not able to speak up for themselves and put forward their case, but for whom the rules have also just been changed.

Imagine the situation in a school for pupils with severe learning difficulties where two children with autism in the class go swimming on a Thursday. It is 1pm in the afternoon on the Thursday and the teacher suddenly says, "We usually go swimming on Thursday but we're not going today as the minibus is broken. We are going to go for a walk instead."

There is no reaction from the two children with autism at first. A few of the others express their sadness and moan. But the teacher goes on to explain what happened to the minibus and that hopefully it would be repaired by next week. They then set off for a walk over the park. As the class begin to walk past the bus towards the school gate the two children with autism get very agitated. One of them begins to scream and bite their arm. The other hits out at the child near to them.

The teacher may be surprised as they didn't seem to bother when they were told about no swimming so she tries to explain again and at length that the brakes are not working and the bus is not safe.

By the end of the afternoon the teacher is exhausted. They never got to the park due to a major incident with one of the pupils with autism.

"but it says in the procedure book..."
"but it says on the timetable that we swim on a Thursday afternoon"
"but it says in my internal diary that we swim on a Thursday afternoon."

The children are not attention seeking, selfish children who are too used to getting their own way. They are children with autism who find it extremely difficult to cope when set rules change. Great anxiety arises within them due to confusion and fear of the unknown.

The teacher may claim that she explained the situation several times, but the children with autism probably had no idea they were being spoken to, let alone what the explanation was about – even if they appeared to, even if one of them echoed, "no swimming today, park instead".

We need to understand this so much more if we are to be able to help these pupils cope in a world where rules do alter, where plans do change. Then perhaps we will be able to set in place the strategies which will help to relieve some of that anxiety and stress. **But first we have to understand.**

Religion – why I am right
It makes little or no difference what religion I am in because I practice them all the same way, my way. Of course I enjoy the correct and exacting enactment of rituals. But one of my favourite aspects of a religion is its set of rules, precepts or commandments. I enjoy keeping them (or rather, my own modified enhanced version of them) perfectly all day, unbroken for the duration of the period of time, while I am intensely interested in that religion. I do this by learning them and repeating them to myself often during the day. I get a lot of enjoyment from this, but I feel very threatened by anyone or anything likely to make me break them. This does make it difficult for me to interact with people not in the religion as well as some people who are supposedly in it. That is about the extent of my 'spiritual life'. I have no experience of 'guidance' or 'influence' or being 'changed' or 'surrender', whatever. I have read a lot on these subjects but I do find the explanations and descriptions go round in circles never describing anything concrete and these things are outside my experience.

For me religion is about self-effort and self control, and control of my world. My keeping of these rules is not out of fear of any punishment or hope of reward either by the force of Karma or by any god. I am unable to understand how such rewards or punishment could possibly work. So for me they don't come into the picture. My practice of religion is between me and me. I'm the lawgiver and the judge. The religion is what provides my ideas for this. Of course I don't punish myself for breaking the rules. That is quite upsetting enough, when I am in a state of intense interest in that religion. (Though in the convent I had to whip myself with a cord plaited whip – once I got over the squeamishness and actually plucked up the courage to do it, I really enjoyed it). I had read beforehand about these medieval practices and had found them very interesting. I could hardly believe that I was actually doing them. It was wonderfully exciting!

Sue comments: This makes me aware of the vulnerability of Paula, though I know she would not see it like that. If you are not able to use intuition, to have a 'feeling' for a situation, but only to obey a hard and fast rule there will be countless situations where you will be vulnerable. The need for us to teach how to deal with 'what ifs', the 'maybes' and the 'it depends' of life leap out at me. These are skills that children develop as they grow and experience life – but not so with the child with an autistic spectrum disorder. For these individuals the predictable, concrete rule or routine is the way life should be. When, for whatever reason, changes occur we need to recognise that stress levels and feelings of anxiety begin to rise. Reasoning, at this stage, is not helpful. In order for the anxiety and stress to be kept at bay we need to help develop an understanding of uncertainty, how to deal with changes and rules that are flexible. I believe this can be done but people don't think to do it and then are surprised by the reaction of the person with an asd over what seems to us neuro typicals a trivial alteration in a day's plan.

When I read the following section I began by feeling rather uncomfortable. Paula has taken quite an emotive and sensitive topic to illustrate her reasons for being right. However, it also helps to see how logically she operates, unaware of what I might consider to be a difficult subject to talk about. Initially, I made virtually no comment on this section but in discussion with Paula she felt I should as others may feel as I do about the subject. Paula does not understand this or think it is valid but she is aware that others are more likely to feel like I do than herself.

Trying to explain the sensitive nature of this subject led me to consider a teenager with autism and learning difficulties I currently work with who, when walking round the supermarket will suddenly ask a passer by, "Why are you so fat?" or burst out laughing in front of someone and say, "You have got a very funny face."

Is this rudeness and insensitivity or is it reality as he sees it, with little ability to sense others feelings, no awareness of the social graces that enable most of us to notice someone who is very overweight, and think about why internally but never say anything?

Read on and see what you think about Paula's view on what I see as a sensitive subject.

Harelip – why I am right
I recently saw a TV programme about a population of people living in a remote area of Pakistan. A significant number of the children were born with the harelip defect. The reason for this, as explained in the programme, is that the population intermarries in order to preserve wealth and other resources within the group. The birth of a child with the harelip is a tragedy for the family, largely because it makes the marriage of the child impossible. In the absence of higher education and training, etc marriage is one of the few things to which one can aspire.

A couple originally from Pakistan have begun a charity which raises money, in order to fund English doctors to go to that area and perform the simple operation to correct the harelip – something that is done automatically in this country. Not every child with the defect is selected for the operation; they must be in good general health. For instance, because of the lack of facilities in which the surgeons have to work, any child with a chest infection would not be operated on, as due to lack of modern equipment they may not survive the anaesthetic. The programme concentrated on about four children. It followed the progress of a girl of about thirteen years of age, who following her operation was transformed into a beautiful young girl. This was hailed as a happy ending because as a result of this in a few years' time she would be able to get married! Well, it may or may not be a happy ending.

Let's consider the various possible genetic scenarios for when she gets married. The gene for harelip within the population is obviously a recessive one, as the prevalence of harelips within the population is explained by intermarriage. So let's consider the girl's genetic make-up for this particular characteristic.

Key   H = hare-lip gene
        N = normal gene

Girl = H H

Now if we take the worst possible scenario, if she marries a boy from the same population who has had the same corrective surgery and they have four children.

His genetic make-up will also be H H.

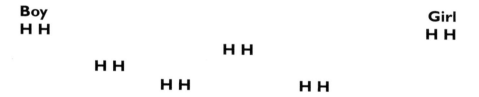

All four children, having the faulty gene from both parents, will be born with harelips.

Supposing she marries a boy from the same population who does not have a harelip but has one faulty unexpressed gene and is therefore a carrier.

Boy
H N

                             Girl
                             H H

H H

H H

N H   N H

Two of their four children have harelips and two do not but are carriers. Supposing she marries a boy who is neither a carrier nor has a harelip, whether from within or outside the population. Now, the scenario is much better.

Boy
N N

         Girl
         H H

N H

N H

N H   N H

None of the four children have harelips but all four are carriers. If these children marry outside the population it is extremely unlikely that they will mate with another carrier, so their faulty gene is unlikely to be expressed. But if they continue with the tradition of marriage within the group the harelip problem will continue. So what is the answer for these people?

1. Genetic counselling? If a test could be done in the early stages of pregnancy to see if the harelip was likely to develop and the faulty foetus aborted, would this be the answer? Well no, because:
   - People of Islamic faith would not accept abortion.
   - Abortion is too extreme a course to take for such a minor defect, which is so easily repaired in rich countries.
   - It would not help much in eliminating the faulty gene within the population if foetuses with one faulty gene, who would therefore not express the harelip characteristic, were not allowed to go full term as they would be carriers.

The best solution would be to persuade this group that the children must marry out to prevent having harelip children. For this to happen the reason for inter-group marriage must be addressed. It was to protect wealth and other resources, by keeping them within the group. Therefore, for progress to be made in the elimination of the harelip in this area, the corrective surgery needs to be backed up by economic development projects and further and higher education opportunities so that girls can have something better to aim for than simply to get married.

Like many things that go wrong in this world the perpetuation of the harelip is largely due to poverty caused by unequal distribution of resources in an unfair world.

Sue comments: Then there are times like with the above example when I think — well Paula you're right!

Chapter 4

Anger, violence and me!

At primary school I was often beaten up when we were put outside in the school yard for break or in the interval between one teacher leaving the classroom and the next one arriving. On one of these later occasions a boy began to hit me. I was not strong enough to fight him off. Then the teacher entered the room and he stopped hitting me. I took the opportunity to bite him and scratch him with my nails. While he did not respond I continued until the teacher dragged me off him. I was punished but I didn't care, I was so happy to see his blood up my nails. When I understood that they would not hit me in the presence of the teacher or any other adult, I used this information to protect myself from further assaults. For instance, in the break times I walked through the playground to the front entrance of the school and stood there. It was near the street with houses and adults going about shopping or whatever. I got into trouble for being there but it was better than being beaten up.

Sue comments: The thing that jumps out at me in this rather disturbing tale is that Paula had no awareness or understanding that the boy would do nothing if the teacher was in the room. The fact that the teacher would get cross with her did not make the slightest bit of difference.

As teachers we expect to be able to be in control and that our presence has an effect upon the children we come into contact with in our role as teacher. This is true in a special school as well but we have had a clear example from Paula that status means very little to her. Certainly, when she was at school she was completely unaware of what kind of behaviour was expected of her once the teacher was around but quickly picked up how the other children responded to the presence of a teacher and used this to what she saw as her own advantage. Telling her off had very little impact as the focus for Paula was the sight of the boy's blood under her nails. This would have been a very tactile as well as visual sensation for Paula as someone with an autistic spectrum disorder. This meant that the words of the teacher – the person with supposed power – were not really heard.

In secondary school, PE or Physical Education class could be very frightening. There was a climbing frame against one wall. Some brave people used to climb right up to the ceiling. I find the idea terrifying. There was also a wooden thing called a horse. The other girls used to run up to it and put both hands on it and somehow jump over it. I couldn't understand where their hands went when they jumped over it. I would have thought they got in the way. I used to run up, put my hands on the horse, jump about three or four inches from the ground and run away again. But PE lessons could be frightening even without equipment.

One terrifying exercise was the backward roll. The teacher told us to lie down on our back on the ground. Then we had to put our legs in the air, put our feet over our shoulder and then stand up. Everyone managed it first time except me. I went as far as putting my legs in the air but I was too filled with fear to go any further. The teacher said, "You will stay in every afternoon after school until you have done the backward roll." So I stayed alone with the PE teacher each afternoon. She continued to demonstrate and explain how to do the backward roll and I continued to whimper in fear, "I can't, I can't, I can't." Then either the second or third afternoon the PE teacher suddenly squatted down in front of me, grabbed my ankles and began to force my legs in the direction of my shoulders. I squirmed and struggled, screaming and screaming. I got free and kicked her very hard in the face with both feet to keep her off me, and then I ran off crying. Next day I was called before the headmistress and was suspended.

Sue comments: The issues here are about being terrified of something that is thought to be quite ordinary and how this meant that Paula was totally focused on her own fear and had no sense of anxiety about kicking the teacher in the face. Can you think, like I can, of individuals with an autistic spectrum disorder who are afraid of the ordinary? My own examples would include a fear of fruit, of buttons, of cameras, of balloons (which led to similar dire consequences for me as a young student teacher many, many years ago). Paula could not understand how anyone could do a backward roll, she was terrified and yet she was forced because it was just an ordinary backward roll.

Twenty five years ago I could not understand that a balloon was a terrifying object and so as an illustration to a story I began to blow one up in class – the dire consequences for me were a severe bite in a delicate part of my anatomy and I had the young woman concerned sent home. After all, it was only a balloon! But, like Paula, that young woman was terrified and when I look back I can see that now. She did not speak but had made it clear to me and I just went on blowing up the balloon and telling her it was "just a balloon" and there was nothing to be frightened of!

If the person with an asd is scared of something we need to know and to grasp that they are really scared. Us giving an explanation of some kind is irrelevant – after all they have a difficulty with our communication anyway so in a state of terror why on earth should we anticipate that some verbal explanation will help the situation – but we do!

I recently became very upset and violent while anticipating a trip to London. Before that I had been quite peaceful and had very few tantrums for some time. I seem to have been growling a bit. One of the reasons is that since September I have been studying Buddhism by distance learning from Exeter University. I was just about keeping up with the course and was reasonably on schedule for my second essay deadline. Life seemed quite sorted out. For me it goes something like this: First I do this and then I do that, afterwards I do that. Like everything seems to be under my control. Then my husband said we had to go to London to see his elderly relative in her nineties. I couldn't see any way of getting out of it. My husband had just had his annual cancer check up and as he was very tired recently there was some more chance he may get sick. Maybe if we didn't go, one of them would die and they would have missed the last chance to meet again. But I absolutely hate going on holiday. I hate to travel on a long journey on the train with someone else. I can't listen to a tape I've made and relax and forget the situation. When someone else is with me I am forced to experience the unpleasant situation. I hate having to share one room in a hotel or hostel or whatever. At home at least I have my own room to go to and relax.

My biggest annoyance was breakfast which used to cause such tantrums. I would then be too ashamed to go to the breakfast room. I would inevitably wake up about 6am while my husband would not be ready for breakfast until 8am or 8.30am. When I tried to be polite and wait for him I ended up having tantrums. Nowadays unless it is a hostel where I can fix myself something I just bring some buns and make some coffee with my mini-jug at 6am or 6.30am and I don't go to the breakfast room at all.

Sue comments: It is not just that Paula likes a plan and to know what is happening, for how long and what will happen next. She needs this to feel secure and to be able to relax. The followers of the TEACCH (Schopler and Olley, 1982) model of working with children who have an autistic spectrum disorder have known this for many years, but how many school children with autism do not know what is happening each moment of the day and who feel totally confused by the things that are said to them? Therefore, they are in a state of panic and feel out of control for a great deal of their time. Then we label them as children with challenging behaviour who go on to be adults with challenging behaviour!

So all of this dread started to play on my mind. Plus the fact that my studies, so carefully planned, would be disrupted. Whereas before I could see a well ordered plan, now I could see only darkness, nothingness. Everything was out of my control now and threatening. I had about three weeks to wait for this trip and my tension grew and grew. At first I had thought it might not be too bad. I would just have to visit his relative and we wouldn't have to stay long and the rest of the time I could hopefully tape or write while Frank was out. Then he insisted we visited a friend of his. Worst of all he found two letters (very old) from two people I knew from a library I had temped at in London. He kept on and on at me to write to them and fix a time to meet. I didn't want to but he kept on and on so finally I agreed. I was informed that one had died but the other woman agreed to meet me. Now it had all reached unbearable proportions. My tension level was sky high. The woman next door saw me in Marks & Spencer a few days before we left. She said my face had been like thunder. I had been shouting in the shop and at home. Finally the day before we travelled, as my husband went on and on about the people I would have to meet, I exploded. I cried and cried and I shouted that before I'd married I'd had my own life and my own home. I'd go out during the day and in the evening could close my door and I didn't have to see anyone until the next day. I had all those hours free. Sometimes people came but they always went away. You never go away. You're always there. I punched him on the head and shoulders and chest and kicked him in the legs (he was sitting down). I continued until I finally lay sobbing on the floor. Next day I was off to London. My mood did not improve until I had a day on my own when I sat for hours in an organic café watching the people and later bought myself an enormous anthology on my all-time favourite subject – consciousness.

During my stay I got up every morning at 6am. It was a hostel so bread and milk was always in the fridge and I concealed jam overnight behind an ornament. I had my breakfast alone and stayed out of the bedroom until about 8am. Then in the evenings I left the room from about 10pm until 12.30pm to sit in the quiet room and write, listen to myself on tape or whatever. When we returned home I was still tensed up and had more tantrums but they did not end in violence.

Sue comments: How true rings the National Autistic Society's slogan for their 40th year anniversary, "The problem is understanding". Paula has been able to develop strategies to prevent her exploding and becoming aggressive with people who do not understand – for most of the time. There are exceptions to this, as we have already heard. However, by keeping to herself and following her own routines she is able to maintain control and stay on an even keel. It is not that Paula does not want to have anything to do with people, quite the contrary if you are meeting to discuss some aspect of Buddhism or the current political situation in a country that Paula has an interest in. What she finds so intolerable is social interaction that is out of her control and with which she can see no purpose and therefore no end, no time limit.

It strikes me that we often impose ourselves on people with an asd who cannot tell us they do not want us around or who are unable to get away from all the other residents who they live with. If, on occasions, they get aggressive for what we see as no apparent reason, maybe we need to give them a little more space and accept their individual needs a bit more. I am not saying that we just leave people with an asd in their own world and make no attempt to make relationships. I think that is a dangerous stance to take and often results in the poor emotional health of the person, an area in which we have been greatly helped to understand (Clements and Zarkowska, 2000). But we should not be surprised at sudden aggressive acts if we are responsible for placing intolerable social pressure on an individual.

Once I went to a social in a church hall just at the bottom of my street when I was about sixteen. A boy about my age offered to take me home. I said "No need, I live in this street," but he would not go away. Then he suddenly dragged me unexpectedly down a side street and began to sexually assault me. I immediately began to tantrum. My teeth clenched, my hands clenched and I began to scream and cry loudly. I dug my nails into his face and scraped them down again and again. He then held my hands and restrained me. I sunk my teeth into his hand and kept biting until he pushed me off. Then I began to scream and cry loudly again. Lights went on in the street. Windows opened. He ran away. A woman came out of one of the doors to ask if I was OK, but I pushed her aside as I ran after the boy still screaming. I had a strong compulsion to bite his other hand but he could run much faster than I could and he got away.

I get annoyed when people assault me like that. I don't wear lipstick or make up or miniskirts or anything to encourage this kind of behaviour. I dislike this kind of contact and want to be alone. Yet it happens occasionally. When it does I always confront the person responsible. Once I was sitting on a bus trying to relax, sitting by myself listening to a tape I had made. But I could not get comfortable, it was like there was a crease or lump in the seat or someone had left something there. I put my finger under my bottom and was surprised to feel another human finger. I turned round and saw a young man seated directly behind me. I immediately shouted at him, "Why are you putting your finger under my bottom? Why are you treating me like this? I am not wearing lipstick or a mini dress or anything to encourage this kind of behaviour. There are plenty of woman on this bus looking like that. Why don't you pick on them?" I shouted after him as he silently got up and walked quickly to the front of the bus and got off at the next stop. Relieved, I put my tape back on again and relaxed for the rest of the journey.

Sue comments: These two events that Paula has described on first reading made me feel sad and think again about how vulnerable she seems in these situations. But then I began to think about how well she handled them and that her response to both those men actually had an impact. The first because she hurt him quite badly and the second because it was on a bus and she cared nothing for what other people might think, she was not embarrassed at all and so she yelled at him until he got off the bus. Often you hear about girls and women being so scared or intimidated they freeze and therefore really suffer, or they are embarrassed and don't like to say anything or ask for help and draw attention to themselves. Thank goodness this was not, and is not, the case with Paula. This is one of the advantages of not being aware of how other people view you.

Once I was waiting alone at the bus stop. A man came along to the stop. He began to talk about the buses. I was annoyed. I didn't know him and it made me feel uneasy. I was just going to put my earphones in to blank him out when things became a bit scary. He asked, "Where are you going love? If you like, I can ring my friends on my mobile and they can come and pick us up in their car." I had to go and stand in a shop to wait for my bus and risk missing it. Then when it came I had to sit beside someone despite the many empty seats available, in case he should try to sit beside me. I was hoping he would get off the bus soon, but he stayed on all the way to town. Then I had to let him off first and start off in some direction so I could be sure he wasn't following me. I was very annoyed. A few days later I went into my local chemist to collect some medicine I had left the prescription for earlier. I was horrified to see him standing at the counter chatting to one of the sales assistants. Then the pharmacist came out from the back with my medicine. "Can you give me your address please," she said as they always do for security reasons. I pointed at the man and said in a loud voice, "I'm sorry, but I can't give you my address while this man is here. He has been bothering me at the bus stop." To my delight he quickly scuttled out of the shop and I was able to give my address and get my medicine.

Sue comments: I feel I want to say – "Well done Paula." I do not think many women would have done that. The honesty with which she faces these very difficult situations has much to teach us.

(The following is repeated in the chapter on my special interest, but it is of relevance to this section as well, so I have included it here.) A lot of my tantrums happen as a result of being blocked in carrying out the demands of my current special interest. For instance when my interest in Buddhism was just about at fever pitch, my husband was depressed. He did not leave the house for two months. When I only went to the corner shop he would be filled with anxiety. I could not go far. So when the Tibetan cookery class I had enrolled on came up I was unable to go. This was important for me at the time because the Buddhist temple I was attending was Tibetan and a big part of lay Buddhist practice is to bring food for the monks, so I really needed to learn to cook Tibetan food. Later when I was able to get out and about again I did attend the class and as usually happens with practical things I learned virtually nothing. But I wasn't to know that then. To me at the time it was just about the most important thing in the world. So during the time when I knew the first session was going on I began to tantrum. I screamed and cried loudly. I banged my head against the wall. I sobbed for about three quarters of an hour until I could hardly breathe and my head was throbbing and I lay exhausted on the floor. I was not however violent towards my husband on that occasion.

Sue comments: Paula writes more about her special interest elsewhere in this book but how important it is for us to understand the all-consuming hold that a special interest can take over the person with autism. For Paula at this time it was Buddhism and not being able to attend this cookery class associated with her special interest caused a major outburst. There was anger at the original realisation but an even more powerful reaction at the actual time the class, that she was unable to attend, was taking place.

We tend to think of a person with a learning disability and a special interest as having an obsession. Ones that spring to mind from my experience are the collecting of receipts or plastic bags or visiting particular shops with televisions in. If these desires are blocked in some way or we say "You have enough plastic bags and you do not need any more," we are often amazed at the passion with which our statement is objected to. Just consider for a moment the reaction Paula has described at not being able to attend her Tibetan cookery class. As Paula, in a later chapter, turns to focus on the nature of special interests in her life and how they arrive without warning and fill her every waking moment, try to think of those individuals you know who have an asd and an additional learning disability. What passions do they have?

Chapter 5

How I sense the world

Seeing

Sometimes I have difficulty in taking in my surroundings in their entirety. If something changes in my environment my mind seems to be fixed in such a way that it overrides my ability to realise that my surroundings have changed.

For instance, I once went for an interview to be on the team for the National Autistic Society's accreditation scheme. On arrival, a young man I knew who also has Asperger syndrome was ahead of me and he went in first for his interview, while I was waiting outside. I felt I needed to go to the toilet. Although I had been to these offices before I could not find the toilet, so I asked the secretary for directions. She said something like, second on the left. Anyhow, I tried to follow her directions. I entered the room and walked towards the far wall where I expected the toilet facilities to be. To my right there should have been first a coat stand and then a bath and to my left a mirror. I did not notice their absence. My vision was concentrating on the far wall. Then I heard someone running and entering the room I was in. The secretary said, "Paula, that's not the right room, can you come out." I suddenly noticed that there was no toilet ahead of me. I don't know when I would have noticed if the secretary had not called me out. I turned around and to my right seated at a table were the Asperger syndrome outreach worker, the young man with Asperger syndrome and a woman I did not recognise. As I took in the scene I gradually realised I had gatecrashed the interview. Later when it was my turn to go in for an interview the outreach worker introduced me to the other woman, "This is Marilyn, who you have already met." "Have I?" I said puzzled. I'd completely forgotten the incident that had just occurred.

When I was working on the review team for the National Autistic Society's accreditation service I had a hotel room to myself with a bathroom ensuite. After hanging something in the wardrobe I found to my horror that the bathroom had disappeared. I kept very still and forced myself not to panic as I thought, "Oh no, not again," because all my life rooms, buildings, whole streets, have disappeared and while taking what I thought was a familiar turning I have found myself in a frightening and unfamiliar world. As I surveyed the hotel room which no longer had any evidence of a bathroom, I suddenly realised that by opening the wardrobe door I had obscured the entrance to the bathroom from my view. So I thought it is OK, everything's OK.

Sue comments: I get lost quite regularly myself and often need to do a route several times to really know where I am going. But to go into a room thinking it is a toilet where there are a group of people, and to carry on into the room and over to where I thought the toilet should be with no awareness of the people, let alone the lack of toilet, is unusual. It seems to me it is the very focused visual ability combined with a lack of social awareness and therefore of people who were not expected to be there that can explain this behaviour Paula describes so well to us.

Recently I was at a local leisure complex. I had to stay there quite a long time because I was waiting to attend an evening meeting in a nearby venue. I had to use the toilet four times. For the first three times, instead of retracing my steps, I continued in the same direction until I reached the bar which should have been the café I started off from. At times like this it's like I am in a tunnel and only able to observe the scene immediately ahead and it takes a few seconds to take in the fact that it isn't what I expected it to be, then turn round and go back. After three times I thought, "I don't have to do this, I'm an intelligent person, and I can crack this." So the next time I went to the toilet I carefully noted the specific posters that were along the wall leading to the toilet, determined to look out for them and follow them in reverse order on the way back. I did that and it worked, but it felt counterintuitive. It's like my brain seems to get fixed or to gather an almost unstoppable momentum, so that when I pop into a shop briefly or use a toilet or buffet counter on a train, it's normal for me to continue on in the same direction. But if I stay about an hour somewhere, like in a café, I can retrace my steps quite easily. It's like that momentum pushing me on in the same direction has worn off.

I have an impulse to walk very fast towards a specific object. I like it when I'm at the beginning of a long straight road and in the centre of my vision there is an object, like a tall building I can focus on. Then I walk really very fast, as fast as possible and see the building getting bigger and bigger. I love it when the distant building seems to rush towards me. It is so exhilarating.

Sue comments: This description Paula gives of such a visually stimulating experience of walking fast towards buildings makes me think about some of the children I know at an autism specific school who love walking. They like to walk fast and for long distances. Their focus has always seemed to me to be on actually walking and that is why they do not see traffic or appear to have road sense. But maybe they are getting a visual stimulus from trees or buildings rushing towards them that overrides traffic. If this is so there are some clear implications for the way we teach road safety and travel training. Paula herself has learnt to always cross at zebra or pelican crossings where there is a routine for her to focus on and follow. There may well be some learning here for those who struggle to teach the concept of road safety to children, young people and adults with an autistic spectrum disorder.

I remember being terrified when my mother had her hair permed, which was about twice a year. She would go from someone with collar length dyed brown hair to someone with short curly grey hair. Her facial features would seem so much bigger; her teeth seemed to stick out like a horse. If she came near me I would scream and scream, "You're not my mother."

Sue comments: The impact of a teacher, parent or carer altering their appearance and that causing difficulties for a person with an asd is not unfamiliar. I have heard a wide range of anecdotal stories about problems caused by changing hair colour or style, shaving off or growing a beard. The point to be made here is that Paula was TERRIFIED. We therefore need to work much harder at preparing people for what may be to us a simple change.

I find that just wearing glasses alters how I look quite dramatically to one young man with asd that I work with. I first became aware of this when he would not speak to me if I had my glasses on, but if I took them off he would acknowledge me. It was as if with them on he did not know who I was. I have worked with him on why I wear glasses for some work and on getting him used to them on or off. He has got used to them and will accept and acknowledge me with the glasses on. However, he prefers them off and I try to respect this as much as I can. I think when we first began to work together I did not wear them and that is his memory of me and therefore how I should be for him to feel comfortable. It is not about pandering to someone's preference of how I look. It is about recognising the importance of the visual for people with an asd and that looking the same is going to make the development of some kind of a relationship a great deal easier for that person.

This is of course true for other senses as well. Let us have a look at what Paula has to share with us about her sense of hearing.

Hearing

I really cannot endure loud TV or radio programmes, such as chat shows, films, soaps, sitcoms, etc. If I'm in the room when one of these noises begins I start to panic. If I am completing a task, like making a cup of coffee with only about half a minute to go, I try to keep calm and get it done. I keep thinking, "I've got to get out of here." I find I can't concentrate on making my coffee or whatever I was doing anymore because those programmes are thinking their thoughts in my mind. If I don't get away soon I will start to scream and scream and swear and growl and snarl. Soon I will be tantruming and crying loudly.

I do like to listen to something I am interested in. For instance I love to listen to the news over and over again, throughout the day. But if someone turns it up too loud I won't be able to hear it. The vibrations, which occur from it being too loud, block out the sound for me while they seem to be able to hear it better.

The sound of my own thoughts bothers me sometimes too. Like when I wake up, my mind will rehearse negative and/or violent thoughts over and over again. I need to get up and put something bearable into my mind. I like to record chapters from books, or whole books, on subjects that interest me and play them back to myself. They sound like my own thoughts do, but unlike my own thoughts they are predictable and under my control.

Sue comments: Here again we have something different about the way Paula senses the world, linking with her need for predictability and to be in control. Paula is able to explain that to us. What about the child who asks the same questions and wants the same monotone answer every time from everyone he/she meets? "Hello, what's your name, my name is . . . and I have got three cats," or "What colour car have you got? What make is it? How long have you had it? Do you have another car?" etc.

This is very much about the need for predictability in order to feel secure but it is also about ensuring that words you don't want to hear and that can be distressing are not said. There is something about the actual 'sound' of the familiar words and not just their predictability that can make the person with an autistic spectrum disorder feel the difference between comfort and pain, between calmness and panic.

The verbal rituals can get boring for us, and the desire to listen to and watch the same video over and over again can seem mind numbing to us. So much so that we may feel we need to eradicate them and I think that is a mistake that leads to cruelty. So much better for us to have an understanding of the way someone hears things in the world and the predictable routines (that may be verbal or mechanical) that give them a sense of calm. Then we can begin to introduce new words and ideas that need to be taught. But first we need to have a receptive learner and so often the power to enable someone to be receptive to both learning and to the acceptance of some changes lies within our hands. Rather than make use of the knowledge and adapt the way we work, we continue to use our own intuition or the way learning works for us!

If there is one thing I hope to come from this joint writing venture of Paula's and mine, it is that people who do not have an asd and yet work with people who do, will learn to think autistically. We can actually apply the knowledge we have gained from the many other able people with autism now writing, to the people with autism who are not able to tell us and describe their world for us – a world that is very different from our own.

I do not mind loud noises if they have no words attached to invade my mind. For instance, the neighbour on one side of me tried to engage me in her campaign to have the neighbour on the other side of me removed from his rented council house. He fixes motor bikes as a job and has to test them before returning them to his customers. One day she said to me, "I really can't stand the noise of those motorbikes day and night. Some of us have written to the council about getting him evicted. We need some more, will you help us?" "But it doesn't bother me in the slightest," I said. She is one door away from the motorbikes while I am right next door and must be bearing the brunt of it. When I am upstairs in my room reading or writing, with earplugs in trying to block out the TV programmes from next door or downstairs in my own house, I often hear the familiar drone of the motorbike and it affords me protection by dulling the sounds of the media coming at me from all directions, including her rock music. "I can't sleep with the noise of the motorbikes," she moaned. "Well get some earplugs from Boots and wear them in bed like I do," I advised.

Sue comments: Different noises have different impacts on people and so much more so for people with an asd. What is important for us to grasp is the powerful way certain noises can impact and make life unbearable for one person may be a tremendous hearing attraction for another person. The wiz and burr of a washing machine can be the source of hours of contentment for one child with autism and be the root cause of fear of the kitchen for another. De Clercq (2001), talks of the need to develop a manual for an autistic child in order for us to understand the way the triad of impairments impacts upon their individual life. I think we need to add to this a sensory manual for each child with an asd if we are to be effective educators and/or carers.

A few nights ago I woke up at about 4.30am and had to go downstairs and make a drink. It turned out that my husband in the next room had woken at about the same time. There had been a noise which I had heard too, despite having earplugs in. "Your hearing is very acute isn't it?" he said. Even during the day he is always amazed how, when downstairs studying each morning, I hear him getting out of bed and can follow the various stages he goes through getting up and have a cup of tea ready for him when he comes down.

I quite like mechanical sounds as opposed to voices. I quite like it on the bus when there are no people talking on their mobiles, then I relax and listen to the sound of the bus's engine, wheels or loose fittings or whatever. I also like the sounds of central heating ticking over when I am up early in the morning sitting, studying or whatever. Following a period of such silence, if someone suddenly speaks to me unexpectedly I am quite shaken and quite often shriek in fear as my heart beats frantically, even when it's just my husband in the house.

I cut my own hair rather than going to the hairdressers. It isn't just because of the many misunderstandings resulting in my acquiring haircuts I'm not aware of having asked for. It's simply the noise of the incessant rock music and the hubbub of talk about TV soaps. When I have been to the hairdressers I ask for a dry cut, or if they won't do that, a wet cut, no finishing. I think the noise overload contributes to my inability to negotiate about the particular style I want cutting. Many times when I am in a mess with dealing with my hair myself, I would like to seek help from a hairdresser but the dread of the noise level puts me off. Similarly when I would like to go for a coffee in town I tend to look for somewhere that won't have the ubiquitous piped music background. The library is safe. Also, I had thought the museum café was a good bet, but one day I had just sat down there when I heard the ghastly clanging of a live pianist. To me the piano is not a musical instrument, the notes differ little in pitch but are simply bang, bang, bang. It should be reclassified into the percussion section. I don't know if that incident was a one off but I have not ventured back there since.

Sue comments: These are very focused thoughts with vision and hearing to match, but Paula can tell us about, and to a certain extent, can control her own environment and the places she visits. This is not the case for many children with autism and a learning difficulty and even more so for adults with autism and a learning difficulty who may live in a group home with several other people. The pain and torture of certain visual and auditory stimulus that Paula describes must make us consider with much greater care what kind of sensory environment we are providing for people – mustn't it?

Sense of smell

As a child I enjoyed the smell of soiled underwear and was upset about being separated from the laundry bag. I hasten to add that's no longer the case! One of my favourite smells is rice cooking. I hate the smell of raw meat or fish, it's associated with blood and fear. My husband likes duck but it's difficult to find a shop selling it. Once I spotted a shop selling luxury meat and fish and decided to get him some duck but when I entered the shop the smell was horrendous. There was quite a queue and as I was going to have to spend some time there I queued up with my finger and thumb closing my nostrils, to protect myself from it. I wondered why the man who served me was rude to me, someone suggested it may have been because I was holding my nose but I would have imagined it would have been a lot worse for him having to stay in there all day.

Sue comments: Seeing the situation from her point of view – how surprised I still am that this is the case and how important to remember just how difficult it is for Paula to consider another viewpoint in any given situation.

I absolutely hate the smell of roasting chicken, again it's like blood and fear, like the smell I used to have as a child when I fell over, which I did a lot! However, not every supposedly bad smell bothers me. Once, in the Buddhist temple I had the task of frying dried fish. I heard the monks mention my name and then my meditation teacher called me over and said, "What do you think of the smell?" I asked, "The dried fish?" He said, "People who have not grown up with it cannot stand it." "Oh," I said. "It's OK, it's a bit like baked potatoes or roasted chestnuts. It's nice." Then a couple of English people who had been for Buddhism class entered the kitchen to get a coffee. "Yuk," one of them said. "What's that horrible smell? What are you cooking?" she choked, and my meditation teacher laughed.

I take a bit of persuading to go to eat in a department store if I have to negotiate the perfume and cosmetic department to reach the restaurant. The smell of the perfume is horrible, again associated with fear, it reminds me of my mother's friends who used to come to visit her after church. They had fur coats, horrible red lipstick which they left on the cups and this awful smell of perfume. I quite like the new natural products which smell of peach or blueberry or whatever and I will spray them on when I have to go out in public but it's a poor substitute for my natural smell!

Sue comments: I am reminded of emerging teenagers who are reluctant to wash and smell clean and fresh to begin with and then soon start spending ages in the bathroom and come out smelling of all sorts of perfumes and deodorants. For Paula there seems to be a very visual association with the smells that she dislikes, the link to her family upbringing and her mother's friends, the reminder of falling over that she did so often as a child and the ensuing smell of her own blood that followed. Here again Paula is not necessarily giving me answers to the many questions I have about other people with autism but she is making me think more diversely and take into account the smells that are encountered and their associations.

Something I can smell is cancer. Before my husband got sick, we stayed at a Quaker peace and healing holiday place. There was a lady there with cancer. I could smell something of her like blood and also at the same time sugary sweet. Some years later I began to smell the same smell of my husband. It even lingered in the room for some time after he left it. I recognised it. After some time he was diagnosed with cancer. When he had some treatment we were told it had been unsuccessful. I wasn't surprised as I could still smell the cancer smell. Following some more radical treatment the consultant said he was completely clear of cancer. "I know", I said, "I can't smell the cancer any more." The consultant asked me what I meant. When I explained he said, "Well do let me know if you smell anything like that again won't you?"

Sue comments: This is a delicate area and I would not try to suggest for one moment – neither would Paula – that she try to diagnose such a dreadful illness by smelling people. However it does help us to see the importance and the different experience that someone with an asd can have in relation to their sense of smell as well as their other senses.

Sense of taste

I do not like chocolate. The taste is OK but the texture in those solid blocks is horrible! I don't know whether to suck it or bite bits off it. It's horrible. However I find that it is OK grated and sprinkled over puddings or melted in the oven in croissants.

I used to manage the filled chocolates with cream inside and just covered in chocolate but recently for about the last year I've been slicing chocolate up in croissants and melting them to try and somehow get through the mounting back log of chocolate.

Sue comments: I am sure I am not alone in thinking – how about giving me your back log . . . a 'back log' of chocolate is a strange concept isn't it? Well clearly not for Paula!

I only like a certain limited range of foods, for instance, banana and yoghurt for pudding. This has been going on for several years. When I buy, for instance, a trifle for my husband he will sometimes ask, "Are you going to have some as well?" "No," I say, "I'm having banana and yoghurt, just for a change!"

I tend to eat the same thing for lunch almost every day. For instance, those offers of two pizzas for the price of one. I can cut each one into four slices and so for eight consecutive days I have the same meal.

Sue comments: For eight consecutive days Paula knows what is coming every lunchtime and the familiarity and sameness is not boring. It rather seems to bring a sense of security that in turn I feel seems to assist that all-important sense of well being. It is not that Paula will not try new food ever, with preparation and planning she will, but in her own home and environment that she likes to control, sameness is more than just a preference, it's an aid to a calm life.

The longer I have the same thing the harder it is to change to something else, even if the something else is something I used to like. For instance, quite recently I only drank milky drinks like instant hot chocolate or flavoured cold milk. I had no drinks whatsoever based on water. During this period Frank asked me to taste a herbal tea he was having. I would have liked to but I couldn't because it was so long since I had had a drink based on water. There seemed to be an insurmountable hurdle or barrier I just couldn't cross. Of course some weeks later I managed to pluck up the courage to reintroduce water based drinks to my diet but it was difficult. In times of stress I seem to become more rigid in my diet, or when I feel insecure or just because I have to go out somewhere. Later I will turn to the familiar cheese and onion pie or some variety of cheese and vegetable pasty. So on really bad weeks it is up to the bakery for a cheese and veg pasty followed by banana and yoghurt day after day after day.

The things I have every day can alter slightly within the same dairy product or fruit and vegetable range. After 53 years I can safely say I'm not going to be eating steak and chips, followed by apple pie and cream every day!

I used to be terrified of hot food like soups or casseroles. I was frightened it would go over me. So I felt safer with cold dry food. I still feel uncomfortable with hot wet food but manage to cope with hot food by having a hot drink first and making myself feel hot like the food. Then it is not such a shock.

Sue comments: These thoughts on food that Paula has shared make me think about the wide range of eating difficulties/differences so many people with an asd seem to have. Once again Paula has not solved those difficulties but she has given me so many new ideas, new ways of understanding why a particular eating pattern has arisen and perhaps some ideas on how to work with that person in relation to the difficulty – or leave them alone! Banana and yoghurt are quite good things to be eating each day after all. The idea of warming up your body with a hot drink in order to be able to eat hot food is something I would never have considered but I have since and how helpful it has been.

The sense of touch

I don't like to be touched by someone else even if I know it is going to happen. It is creepy. I cannot feel their hand as I would feel my own. When, for instance, I put my hand on my opposite shoulder inside my sweater to warm my hand I can feel both my shoulder and my hand. But when someone else touches my shoulder I can't feel the hand, only my shoulder, that's creepy.

I particularly dislike someone touching me when I am eating. Eating feels invasive and touching is certainly invasive. Two invasive events at the same time is really too much.

Sue comments: Eating feels invasive! This is something I have not heard before and may well help us to understand how some people with an asd have such difficulties with food. We have explored this a little when Paula talked about her sense of taste but this gives us another dimension to consider with difficulties over food. It is not just how the food might look or taste but the sensation of it entering the body can also feel unpleasant and invasive. If that was the case we might make more effort to try and ensure that the surroundings someone is eating in are as relaxed as possible! Yet I know that for so many children with autism and a severe learning difficulty, the school dining hall is the place where they encounter food and it is a place of noise, busyness and even chaos at times. This can be equally true of the canteen in a day centre for adults with learning disabilities.

I have a lot of difficulty with physical contact. I have never successfully had my eyes tested. I will look through the frames and get a prescription for glasses which I cannot bear to wear because of the increased clarity of seeing things in too much detail, which is overpowering. So I just find my way round without glasses. To get the first part of the eye test done is possible if I hold the frames in place and can be in control. But I cannot manage to have the light shone in my eyes or the test for glaucoma. It is too terrifying.

I'm missing many teeth because of not feeling able to allow the dentist to treat me. However this is better now.

I am quite scared of some people's eyes. I remember I had a doll whose eyes got damaged and that caused me to scream a lot. But some people's eyes scare me as they seem to have gaps between their eye sockets and I get frightened if I am supposed to look at them directly.

Sue comments: We know eye contact can be difficult for many people with an asd and there are several accounts of different reasons for this. Actually being frightened of the look of someone else's eyes is new to me but again how much we have to learn. Eye contact for us 'neuro typicals' is so crucial for relationships and communication. We find it very difficult to operate in another way – but maybe we need to learn how to. I was at a conference recently when a young man with an asd wanted to ask me some questions. As I was about to answer him he turned to look at the floor and explained to me that he needed to focus on the floor if he was going to have any chance of understanding my reply. He said that the range of facial expressions I gave and my increased body movements when I spoke was very confusing for him.

Standing still and speaking in a monotone as well as decreasing our verbal output would all be helpful for communication with many people with an asd. I know that, but the knowledge does not seem to help me remember very well. Without the knowledge in the first place there would be no hope of our communication improving.

I suppose I have quite a horror of my body. I remember my mother used to cut my finger nails because of the horrible feeling of my exposed finger tips making contact with paper, stair rails, things I have to pick up. I now just let my nails grow and break off.

Sue comments: How many times have you, like me, been involved in cutting hair, cutting finger nails, showering someone who hates it – does this expression of what it is like for Paula alter your attitude to the tasks? I know it does mine.

I cannot understand how people wear denim jeans. The material is so hard and stiff, like canvas luggage. I have soft denim material skirts that I wear most of the time when I am not going out. I like a skirt as there is less contact of the material to my body than there is with trousers.

Needless to say I am not very pleased when people touch me if I am not expecting it. I got in to trouble on a nursing course when one of the patients I was alone with in a private room touched me and I screamed loudly. I can't understand why anybody would want to do something like that. I don't understand why people want to touch each other. It is understandable if you are washing a patient or giving other kinds of medical treatment or, for instance, if someone is trying to have children. But I cannot understand why people would want to touch each other for no apparent reason. It is like the way they go to watch silly films about non existent characters and then buy the video and watch it over and over again. What is the purpose of that? Touching is similarly meaningless.

Sue comments: Since I got to know Paula she has taught me a great deal. But there are times when we just have to admit defeat in trying to understand what the other thinks and feels about something. On this issue we feel very differently. I think it is important that I know how Paula feels about the issue of touch but there is part of me that feels very sad. There is a danger here that I am just placing my own set of values on her experience and that is not right or fair. However, I suspect this feeling of sadness is one many parents of children with an autistic spectrum disorder experience if for their child the sense of touch is as abhorrent as it is for

Paula. For a child to not want to be cuddled or comforted in a physical way is extremely hard to grasp – but this is what Paula is trying to explain and the least we can do is listen and respect that. Then move on in the relationship and find new ways of showing that we care, of offering help and support in times of upset. It will seem strange but I can only say that it can also be rewarding.

Chapter 6

The special interest

In this chapter I will try to explain how the special interest begins, how it ends, how it can be in some ways life-enhancing and the compulsive down side of it. For this I am using my own subjective experience. As we know, subjective experience can be notoriously unreliable as a method of investigation, so I am backing it up with anecdotal evidence.

Sometimes when I am answering questions, after having given a talk, someone will ask, "How do you choose which special interest to follow?" I have to explain to them that there is no element of choice in it. Rather there seems to be a vacuum in my mind, so that if I read about some subject or hear someone talking about it, without warning, my mind hones in on some particular aspect of that subject and then expands to cover every detail of it. So I am driven to follow it up. This isn't something I deliberately do, I'm not even aware that it is happening, but soon all my abilities, resources and waking hours are taken up with that interest. While I am not conscious of this happening it just seems like ordinary life.

Before diagnosis and attendance at the Asperger syndrome group, I did not have the concept of 'special interest', I just thought that what was happening to me was ordinary life. So for most of my life special interests have just dragged me along in their wake and then just left me exhausted and burnt out. Recently I've tried to understand how they start. I'm using for this investigation a special interest I had in Mahatma Gandhi. In the late sixties I was invited to a demo against the war in Vietnam. There was a wide variety of literature available about various famous political or peace figures such as Marx, Martin Luther King and Mahatma Gandhi. I focused on Gandhi, then I got something out of the library about him. Then I wanted to know everything about him, have everything he had written and practice everything that he taught. Looking back I realise that the others continued to demonstrate against the war using Gandhi's tactics where appropriate while I was off on a tangent. Having acquired the address of a yoga ashram in India, leaving my possessions, I took a one way ticket to India and was soon shaven-headed and robed as a Hindu nun studying yoga. After six or seven months and having dysentery I got repatriated to England. After recovering, I again gave away my things restricting myself to three changes of clothes and spoke to people about Gandhi, vegetarianism especially promoting pure vegetable soap, only available from Oxfam. During this period my detailed knowledge of Gandhi's ideas enabled me to speak at a Gandhian conference at Greenford.

Sue comments: The feeling of exhaustion is what comes over me when I hear Paula talk about this. It also turns my mind to some of the children and young people I know who seem to incessantly do the same things over and over again unless they are given something else to fill a vacuum of time that they find acceptable. The need to know what is happening and to be in control in some way is a very strong driving force. It seems that if left totally absorbed by that strong driving force it can become quite destructive and debilitating. However, it does not have to be like that. The challenge for those of us working alongside those who are consumed with a passion for something is to understand it first and then to see if it can be used, channelled, contained. All of which leads us to a TEACCH approach (Mesibov and Howley, 2003) as a way of working with children, young people and adults with an autistic spectrum disorder. But how often is this not done, not even understood? We really do have to increase the awareness of autism with professionals working in the field of learning disability.

"It is important to recognise the implications of both the autism diagnosis and the sld when determining special education needs." (Jordan, 2001)

However, while employed in a factory office, I took my Gandhian principles to their logical conclusion by using the workers' toilets rather than the staff one and informed a union representative of the bosses' plans to pay off some workers resulting in the threat of a strike. I was not kept on in that job. A Hindu friend got me involved in helping the homeless and through this I realised that the nuns' order of Mother Theresa of Calcutta was based on the Gandhian way of life. She had taken many ideas from Gandhi especially the wearing of the homespun cloth (Khadi), so big in Gandhi's campaign for home rule. So, after some voluntary work with them I joined the order for 1½ years. This episode did not always go smoothly. As a novice I was put to work washing the clothes in the men's home by hand, with a newly professed nun who had about one week to wait before beginning her new career working in a convent in France. We were not provided with soap bars, only powder, so to tackle the stains I added some cold water and whipped up lots of soap bubbles in the sink. This seemed to infuriate the nun. After about three days working with me she shouted, "Why don't you take a plane and go home." I ran to the office to the head nuns and screaming and crying, I told them, "She told me to take a plane and go home, I don't have to, do I?" I shrieked. They sent for her and told her that if I lost my vocation because of her it would be serious for her. So for the few remaining days, when we worked together she always smiled and said, "Now why don't you make your nice bubbles".

My interest in Gandhi hasn't really finished, I still have a lot of his writings and at times of uncertainty will record them and play them to myself and when you enter my front room you will see a big picture of Gandhi complete with candles and incense.

Sue comments: The security of the familiar, the calming influence it can have. Do we recognise that enough? Do we use that knowledge?

Soon after moving house we had a man from my husband's Quaker meeting to visit us. He explained about his rebellion against his strict religious upbringing and his decision to join the more easy-going Quakers. I found this fascinating and questioned him avidly about the beliefs and practices of the religious group he had left. Feeling the urge to know more I searched the phone book and found an obscure small sect of this persuasion, which I then attended and soon became absorbed in its ethos. I bought the Bible on tape, both Old and New Testament, in the authorised version and played them to myself over and over again. Not satisfied with that I got a Bible reading plan and every day recorded on my Dictaphone the suggested selection of readings. I got up at about a quarter to six in the morning to get it done and played it over and over again to myself during the course of the day. If anything happened to prevent this, like my husband getting up early before I had completed the taping, it resulted in severe tantrums and sometimes violence on my part.

Sue comments: The need to follow through her own plan without interruption or explanation is powerful and can mean that Paula will completely disregard not only someone else's needs but their basic human rights as well!

Within about six months I knew more about what the Bible contained than the people who had been brought up in this system and could answer questions that came up in the Bible study. The first time I answered an obscure question in the Bible study it was a cause of amazement. My bus usually brought me to the church too early and so I got involved in preparing the tray for refreshments. My obvious difficulty in putting out the tray, for instance 10 cups, saucers and spoons plus coffee and sugar, etc was evident to whichever church member was working with me. That person probably assumed that I had a very low intellect, as is the case when people first see me struggling with a practical task without having a chance to talk to me or read something I have written. So when I gave the correct answer it caused a stir. I think they thought it was some kind of miracle. I became involved in outreach work and also voluntary work one day a week in the mission book shop. I have several boxes of books from there as I became very fascinated by the difference between the Calvinist approach (a limited atonement for the chosen few who have to have it whether they want it or not and cannot lose it), and the Wesleyan approach, an atonement available to all but you have to ask for it and you can lose it.

The Christian shop was frequented by members of different denominations and sects and many theological arguments ensued. In these cases I could usually dig up the appropriate verse to prove or disprove anything. Once, a frequent customer of the shop fired a series of obscure questions at me, such as, "Who was Paul's teacher?" When I fired the correct answers back just like a reflex he was astounded. "I've never met a woman who knew her Bible like that," he said. Of course it was easy for me, he only read the Bible, I had recorded it on tape and had been listening to it on the bus that morning. I gave my trendy outfits away to a charity shop, acquired (mostly second hand) more conservative outfits and gave money to missionary work. My mind was completely taken over, usually just repeating silently the Bible quotes I'd taped for that day. The good side was I didn't let my mind wander and rehearse negative or aggressive thoughts. I was relaxed and happy and the people in the church were happy with me.

Then one Sunday a man came to speak in the church. He mentioned the immense age of the earth, this brought up to my mind memories of the physics/cosmology, etc I had studied privately, the findings of which were in conflict with the beliefs of this group. So the whole thing suddenly unwound, it was over. It had gone from the all stage to the nothing stage. I was suddenly repulsed by the beliefs and the clothes. I had some new things to wear, I didn't go back to the church or the voluntary work and didn't bother to try to contact anyone to explain why. For me it was over. People from the church contacted me, at first they were nice then someone got angry but I just didn't bother with it again.

I started to attend the Asperger syndrome group and was introduced to the concept of the special interest by one of the Autistic Society staff who was helping with the group. He kept stressing the need to get away from the all or nothing aspect of the special interest and follow a 'middle way'. He used this phrase rather a lot and I remembered it from when I had studied comparative religion by post, so I asked him if he was a Buddhist, he said he wasn't. However, about this time I saw a TV programme about Buddhism which brought to mind more of what I had learned about it, so I began to attend meditation classes at a Buddhist Temple. Then of course the whole pattern was repeated again.

Sue comments: I feel like saying at this point, are you exhausted yet? You soon will be!

The giving away of things, donating money, buying books, mind filled with repeating the chanting, etc began again. My approach was I suppose novel. The other meditation students helped by offering lifts to the monks, etc but I had read that in the villages in Buddhist countries, ageing householders like myself went to the temple to clean and cook for the monks. I turned up, announcing I was going to clean the place and brought some badly cooked Tibetan food, attempted from a cookery book. The monks were quite pleased and at least tasted whatever food I had brought. Soon I was answering the door and showing people around the temple as though I had been there for years. I guided westerners who had been Buddhists for years through the ritual complexities of offering food and other gifts to the monks. In meditation class during chanting in Sanskrit, the scriptural language of Mahayana Buddhism, I continually had to point out the page numbers to the others who had been coming for years, as they floundered unable to find the place. Once, when I came late I astounded the meditation teacher by chanting the Sanskrit without access to a book. Of course, it was very easy for me, I had been up morning after morning, recording the whole chanting book on my Dictaphone. Although I had by now learned the concept of the special interest it never occurred to me that Buddhism was my latest special interest, for me it was just life.

A lot of my tantrums happen as a result of being blocked in, carrying out the demands of my current special interest. When my interest in Buddhism was just about at fever pitch my husband was depressed. He did not leave the house for about two months. When I only went to the corner shop he would be filled with anxiety, so I could not go far. So when the Tibetan cookery class I had enrolled for came up, I was unable to go. This was important for me at the time because the Buddhist Temple I was attending was Tibetan and a big part of lay Buddhist practice is to bring food for the monks, so I really needed to learn to cook Tibetan food. Later when I was able to get out and about again I did attend the class and as usually happens with practical things, I learned virtually nothing, but I wasn't to know that then. To me at that time it was just about the most important thing in the world, so during the time when I knew the first cookery session was going on I began to tantrum. I screamed and cried loudly, I banged my head against the wall, I sobbed for about three quarters of an hour until I could hardly breathe, my head was throbbing and I lay exhausted on the floor. I was not however violent on this occasion.

Sue comments: An indication of just how very important particular things can be for Paula, but she is not always able to explain this at the time. There are a number of experiences I could recount when someone with an asd has displayed extremely challenging behaviour and I am unable to work out what it is about. They are unable (even if they have some verbal skills) to explain or tell me how they feel and why. But a sense of frustration builds up and bursts. How are we to know? What can we do? Two particular things spring to mind from the experiences that Paula describes.

First, to be very observant and try to ensure we know what is important to the individual with an asd that we are working with. If the small object they have been holding goes missing and as a result their frustrations burst, the situation will be greatly alleviated if we have been aware of the growing significance of the particular small object. We may even have noticed where it was dropped or have ensured there is a spare one to hand so that we are able to prevent the frustrating experiences occurring in the first place.

Second, where possible, it is important to help the young person with an asd learn to understand their own feelings and how to talk about them. This does not develop easily but what an important skill to include within the curriculum. We know the whole area around the understanding of emotions and then controlling them is difficult but how much time do we put into helping them learn this as a skill?

I was so into Buddhism when I went on an accreditation review team. We were based in a hotel and a full moon occurred during the review. At full moon Buddhists can take another three precepts, one of which is not to lie on a high bed. In distress about this I approached the team leader who had the hotel staff prepare a small mattress on the floor at the foot of my bed. Following this, one of the team asked me what my special interest was, another team member answered for me that it was Buddhism. So they began to question me about my practice in terms of it being a special interest, causing me to see it that way too. Of course, the result of that was it completely wiped the whole of Buddhism from my mind. I was finished with it and had no further interest. When I didn't attend for a month the meditation teacher called me up constantly. Once, during that period of one month my husband persuaded me to go and accompanied me to my meditation teacher's birthday. I was offhand and couldn't wait to get out of the place.

There had been an important change, for the first time on that review team I had been openly acting publicly as a person with Asperger syndrome and I had discussed the current details of my life as being a special interest. I thought, yes, Buddhism was just a special interest and then I understood for the first time that all my other involvements, Gandhi, the Ashram and the convent had all been special interests too. I thought, what next? Before long I'll probably be absorbed in something else 100%. Can I really go on like this for the rest of my life? Meanwhile all the effort, money and work I have put into Buddhism will be wasted.

For the first time I realized that I might be hurting people too. For me it is nothing, I don't care. But I suppose if you show a lot of interest in people and shower them with gifts and then suddenly disappear it can be puzzling, even upsetting for them. So I thought to myself, I am not going to let this pattern repeat itself over and over again and dominate me, I'm going to be in control from now on. So I told them I can't be involved to the extent I was before, but I'll come about once a week just to keep up the contact. But I wasn't very confident. While I had been obsessed I had outstripped other people in reverence for the monks, in mindfulness, etc in fact the ethos of the group. Because no-one, no matter how talented and accomplished, for whom that interest is just one of many in a rich and varied life, can ever compete with someone, however handicapped for whom that interest is the only thing that matters in life. Slowly I became able to replicate some of the achievements by my own efforts that had occurred naturally when I had been obsessed. My meditation teacher repeated several times "You seem like yourself again. For a while you were like a different person," he seemed to be bothered about that. Sadly, one of the worrying aspects of all this is the ability to create a kind of 'ideal person'. I mean, of course, ideal only in that ethos or belief system, a person of whom people become very fond perhaps, but a person who no longer exists and cannot be resurrected once the special interest goes from the all stage to the nothing stage.

Recently I have been studying Buddhism by post from Exeter University. Unlike the temple-based Buddhism class, the Exeter course has had a further negative effect on my interest in Buddhism. On two consecutive essays, I have had to follow similar ground, tracing the origins of the basic doctrines, of course I had not considered these doctrines to be true in the sense that scientific findings are true. They are not testable, verifiable or replicable and one cannot carry out clinical trials on them, but they were interesting concepts. But now they had gone from an interesting theory to uninteresting fiction, for me, if something is untrue I find it difficult to engage with it. As my interest in Buddhism waned I observed the void being filled by consciousness (an old favourite), then biology and evolution of the physical organ the brain, broadening to evolution in general.

The evolution aspect of this may have been triggered by a phone message I took on behalf of my husband, from one of his friends who spoke enthusiastically about her grandson who had a place either at Oxford or Cambridge to study natural history. She later phoned again to give the same message to my husband and then the two of us discussed it. A seemingly trivial event like this can be enough to hurtle me into a short lived exhausting episode. Consequently, when I arrived in the city centre to catch another bus to my Buddhism class in the temple, having about twenty minutes to spare, I compulsively dashed into the science floor of the bookshop in town. I eagerly scanned the contents and indexes of books on neuroscience, evolution, etc and scanned interesting chapters. I somehow lost a sense of time and about two and a half hours passed. It was only the sudden awareness of extreme tiredness accompanied by aches and pains that alerted me to the fact that I had been standing in the bookshop for so long and had missed the class. So I had to go for some refreshments instead and catch the bus home. I repeated this behaviour on two further Saturdays, again missing the class.

The next week I finally made it to the class three quarters of an hour late after a shorter compulsive stint at the bookshop. During this period I joined a course on evolution at Birmingham University, bringing my number of courses for this year to four. I am unable to control the number of courses I join per year as they are directly linked to my special interests and as such are compulsive. At the beginning of the year I got a place on the Open University course, 'Religion in Modern Britain' and was in the process of taping all of the course material before the course started, my usual method of study, when my direction was changed by my being asked to teach English to an important elderly monk from India. All my energies now went into reversing a Teach Yourself Tibetan book for English people into a Teach Yourself English book for Tibetan people and holding my language classes, so the religion course was abandoned. During this period I joined a Teaching English as a Foreign Language course but did not feel able to continue with it because of the stringent practical assessments. I then joined the Exeter University Buddhism course followed by the Evolution course. Four courses in one year is not unusual for me although I complete very few of them because either the associated special interest dies a death in which case I may be the most enthusiastic student at the beginning of the year and drop out halfway through, or I may be simply overwhelmed by the pressure of multiple essay commitments.

In the early morning and late evening I've been compulsively taping from books on genetics evolution and fossils. I've had my essays returned from Exeter University with good grades but have been unable to complete the next essay. I have all the notes prepared in their appropriate sections answering the essay question, but every time I pick up the file I am repelled by the now, to me, nonsensical nature of the ideas. I just can't bring myself to write it up. Another special interest has gone from the all to nothing stage. It's almost as if the compulsion not to engage with Buddhism is now as strong as the one that originally drove me into it. During the time I hadn't been attending the Buddhism class I spotted my meditation teacher alone in the city centre. Normally I would have been thrilled to speak to him about Buddhism. Instead I watched him from the entrance to a shop, then I tried to slip down a side street out of sight to avoid him. I remember doing the same thing a few years back after I had just left the Christian Sect; diving down a side street to avoid a former associate from the Christian Shop. I just seem to helplessly repeat the same behaviour over and over again, as if I am programmed. It's like I am some lower animal performing its repetitive behaviour pattern over and over again without much self-knowledge.

Of course, running alongside these 'intellectual' special interests there are those merely on the level of collections of items. I have already touched on this subject when referring to the set of coffees in my first talk and article (Hirsch, 2001).

One such short-lived and very negative special interest began when a woman asked me to take a few products from a postal cosmetic company so she could get free gifts for herself by introducing a new customer. Unfortunately they sent me a book describing liposomes, those fatty spheres which can transport water into the deeper levels of the skin. Soon I was going to Boots the Chemist, reading the different ingredients of the creams, buying the different kinds, not to use them but to have them and learn about them. I was moved on, presumably by a store detective, for loitering so long in front of the expensive creams. I have a tallboy, the drawers filled with different categories of creams, carefully stacked and labelled but completely inaccessible to me because the room and entrance are blocked off by the newspapers, etc which my husband collects. The compulsive side of this I can illustrate. I was trying to complete an assignment for some studying I was doing by post, when the order form from the company arrived. My mind became completely dominated with trying to choose exactly the right price of products to get the free gifts and to complete the sets I already had. This exhausted me mentally making my study impossible. I was happily released from this special interest when the box arrived with the wrong product, a boring shower gel. I was very upset because my sets of face-creams could not be completed as expected, I was fortunately not interested in beginning a collection of shower gels. I hate showers! So I never had anything to do with that company again.

My ongoing interest of this nature is school cardigans. The number of school cardigans I have in black, grey, navy, burgundy and green are each in double figures, with a couple in royal blue and none in red which is too bright. I usually buy from different club catalogues their particular version of the school cardigan in all the colours I like, not all of them offer it in all the colours, so I search the school uniform stalls in market places to fill the gaps in my collection. I was discussing this interest with Sue Hatton who I am writing the book with. She said "You have enough school cardigans." "Yes" I said. Soon afterwards my doorbell rang, it was the postman delivering a package of school cardigans, we had to laugh. Next time I saw her she asked if I had managed to stop acquiring school cardigans. There has been a steady flow of delivery men, I had to admit.

So you have a special interest which comes unexpectedly, unsought, virtually unnoticed, filling every aspect of your life. It's thrilling, exhilarating, as driven by the urge for completeness, you strive to know everything there is to know about it, acquire everything associated with it, practice every aspect of it. The end, when the special interest goes from the all to nothing stage is similarly unsought and seems to happen when the interest proves to be incomplete or incompleteable as for instance if religious ideas prove to be untrue in a concrete sense. Of course, the capacity is still there, ready to be filled seemingly arbitrarily by whatever else gains entry to the void vacated by the previous interest. On the one hand the special interest is enabling. It seems to lend talents or uncover and use talents not accessible in ordinary life, but it does make ordinary life difficult. Any possessions or comfortable life you have built up may be sacrificed because you have to have everything associated with that special interest. You have to know everything, do everything, buy everything to do with it. The down side is that it is so compulsive. It fills your mind so it is difficult to think about anything else and if something or someone stands in your way of carrying it out there will be tears and tantrums to the point of exhaustion and sometimes violence. So, I've tried to explain the special interest as I experience it. The special interest may seem like a burden, but it has enabled me to experience success, when the only alternative has been failure and rejection in the non autistic world.

Sue comments: Getting to the end of this chapter could make you feel very tired but what Paula has tried to do is share that feeling of being driven by an interest to the point of exhaustion. She has also tried to point out some of the valuable aspects of having a special interest. It gives her purpose and meaning. It offers routine and plans for the day, the week, the month, etc. It helps her to feel secure in the pursuit of more information on something she likes and knows a considerable amount about already. It also gives her the opportunity for meeting people, for interacting and for taking part in a certain section of the community. People are important to Paula and help give her a sense of well being and to boost her self esteem. This emotional well being is something that we need to take greater account of with those people with an asd who cannot express themselves in a way we easily understand. We need to find ways of being with them, and alongside them, that are acceptable and to help develop an enjoyment in human companionship. With an increased understanding of asd we can begin to do this on the terms of the person with an asd and slowly introduce other aspects of relationship to them. The 'special interest' also creates a great opportunity for learning and Paula is not only good at learning, she enjoys it and it strengthens her sense of well being even further.

I think with children and young people with an asd there is a greater understanding of the special interest and a tolerance, but as yet have we really found ways of using it as an effective learning tool? The TEACCH model (Mesibov and Howley, 2003) has taught us to see the special interest as a reward and a tool to get the child or young person to do something from our agenda in order for them to then follow their own agenda – Thomas the Tank Engine, helicopter drawing, Disney cartoons. But there may be much more we can do and the building up of self esteem is crucial for the well being of so many children, young people and adults with an autistic spectrum disorder.

The Conclusion

Draw your own conclusions. What I have shared won't give you the answers to all the questions you have about different people but it might help. The experiences of writing and speaking about myself since I got my diagnosis has helped me understand myself more. I have learnt to work with my Asperger syndrome and cope. I think it is important to be clear about what you can and cannot do. I can't cross roads because I do not understand what the cars are doing, what they can do or what they are supposed to do, but ask me about theories around reincarnation and I could talk for hours.

It is interesting when I talk to people about my Asperger syndrome that they always laugh in the same places, not at the times I expect them to laugh but now I know the laugh is coming and can wait for it even though I do not see the situation as funny.

It has been liberating to be honest. I would rather people know than try to cover up and if my being honest can help others in the way Sue seems to think it can, that is a good thing and makes the struggle I have had in life seem a little more worth it!

Paula Johnston

I want to return for a moment to the story Paula began the book with about Paula attempting to look like her peers and the incident with the car and the parking ticket. When the woman first asked Paula to watch her car she said "Yes" but also commented that this was said without any understanding. I highlight this at the end of our story because it is the key those of us who work with people who have the label of asd and sld need to grasp and respond to. Paula has a very high IQ and yet there is so much about the world that she does not understand without a considerable amount of help. So I conclude with a plea to all those staff who work with the children, young people and adults that I am concerned about here – so often they do not understand what on earth is going on and yet without thinking we alter a routine, give an explanation or show a new picture/symbol and then wonder what the problem is when their behaviour becomes difficult to manage or they do something we did not expect. The slogan of the National Autistic Society in their 40th anniversary year "The problem is understanding" needs to be taken to heart – but the problem is not just our understanding. We first of all need to grasp that the person with an asd so often does not understand what we say or do and unlike Paula they are not able to tell us in a way that we can comprehend!

> "What happens now Sue? Usually when you give me a lift home you get out of the car and come into the house and we look at the calendar, but you are not getting out of the car!"

> "Oh sorry Paula, I do that in order for us to sort out when we are next meeting but we already know that as we agreed it earlier on and put it on the calendar, so I don't need to come into the house, but I can if you want me to?"

> "No, it is just that I did not know what was happening as you had not explained and you were doing something different."

Sue Hatton

Postscript

Paula:

I am not sure if I want my name to be on the book. I don't feel I want people to think it is me who wrote it anymore.

Sue:

Why is that Paula? I thought you were pleased to be able to help other people who are trying to work with those who have an asd and learning difficulties who so often do not understand some behaviour and do not know how to work effectively. Your insights give us so much more to think about and consider. They have helped me on so many occasions think differently and therefore more creatively about some of the children at the school and what their behaviour might be telling us.

Paula:

Yes, that is good but the thing is when I read the words now and read them out to people when I am giving a lecture, it no longer sounds like me. It sounds like an exaggerated version of me. The words are true, the things all happened, but I feel quite different now.

All the writing about it, all the speaking to different people has helped me to understand myself and my Asperger syndrome so much more. This has meant that my life is not the catalogue of disasters that it used to be. I feel more in control and more able to understand the world about me. That made it not feel right to have my name on the book.

Sue:

That is very interesting and such a valuable insight Paula, it makes me want to include it towards the end of a book – perhaps in a postscript. I work with a number of young people trying to help them understand their own asd and I often talk to staff and parents about the importance of children and young people being told that they have an asd and what all that means. I believe this helps and can give meaning and understanding to the confusion and alienation they so often feel. Your very experience of re-

reading all you have written and now feeling that you have moved on from that experience will help to confirm the value of telling children and young people so they are able to have some understanding, even if that understanding is limited. I feel strongly that developing self awareness is very important and that it can help raise self esteem – something so important for all human beings and often at a low level for people who have an asd. What you are saying is that the whole experience of writing the book has developed your self awareness and enabled you to feel more at ease in the world... at least I think that is what you are saying.

Paula:

Talking about the Asperger syndrome in public to different groups has helped me to talk about it openly to people where I do my voluntary work. For instance, this means instead of trying to cover up and dread something going wrong, I have actually got over that. Leila, the woman I work with in the library says things like, "Well, you say you have got this syndrome but you seem normal to me." But when I show a lot of energy, for instance when moving piles of books, she admits that I am unusual and maybe it is due to my Asperger syndrome. This is the kind of thing that can make me reluctant to talk about it openly when people say something good about me, like that I work harder than other people and am more willing to do what I'm told. If I say, "That's because I am autistic," it spoils it for them. It is something nice for them if it is an attribute respected in a religious culture.

I've got to say that I haven't had a tantrum for ages now, partly because talking about how it begins, or what happens just before it, or what brings a tantrum on, really helps me to recognise the danger signals and to avoid it happening. That is a really good thing.

Sue:

That's just great and again confirms what I feel about some of the young people I work with. If they can be helped to understand what makes them angry and lash out, they too can learn to handle feelings which take control.

You've helped me so much in my work, Paula – thank you. It is good to know you have benefited from the process of writing this book as well. Thank you for sharing your life experience with me and all who read this book.

References

Clements, J. and Zarkowska, E. (2000) *Behavioural concerns and autistic spectrum disorders – explanations and strategies for change*. London: Jessica Kinglsey Publishers.

Cumine, V., Leach, J. and Stevenson, G. (1998) *Asperger syndrome. A practical guide for teachers*. London: David Fulton Publishers.

De Clercq, H. of Opleidingscrentrum Autisme (Belgium). When talking at a conference in Hereford in 2001. The conference was called "Collaboration between parents and professionals".

Jones, G. (2002) *Education provision for children with autism and Asperger Syndrome – Meeting the needs*. London: David Fulton Publishers.

Hatton, S. (2002) A summer outing for Tom's circle of support. *Good Autism Practice Journal*, Volume 3, Issue 2, 72–74.

Hirsch, P. (2001) A day in the life of . . . *Good Autism Practice Journal*, Volume 2, Issue 1, 7–11.

Jordan, R. (2001) *Autism with Severe Learning Difficulties*. London: Souvenir Press.

Mesibov, G. and Howley, M. (2003) *Accessing the curriculum for pupils with autistic spectrum disorders. Using the TEACCH programme to help inclusion*. London: David Fulton Publishers.

Schopler, E. and Olley, J. G. (1982) Comprehensive educational services for autistic children: The TEACCH model. In: Reynolds, C. R. and Gutkin, T.R. (eds) *Handbook of social psychology*. New York: Wiley.

Other autism resources published by BILD

Supporting a Child with Autism: A Guide for Teachers and Classroom Assistants

Sharon Powell

This pocket booklet provides a practical introduction to autism for teachers, classroom assistants and other support workers. It includes plenty of examples of the sorts of behaviour that a child with autism may show in the classroom, followed by a guide to developing effective strategies for working with a child with autism.

The booklet finishes with a question and answer section on some of the trickier situations you may encounter.

2002 £1.80 BILD members £2.00 full price ISBN 1 904082 39 4

Positive Approaches to Supporting People with Autistic Spectrum Disorders

John Brooke

A workbook and assessment booklet for staff who are working through the optional units of the LDAF Certificates in Working with People with Learning Disabilities at levels 2 and 3.

By studying the text and working through the activities, staff will gain an understanding of:

- the triad of impairments
- the autistic spectrum
- behaviours characteristic of autism
- meeting the challenges of communication
- meeting the challenges of interaction
- meeting the challenges of imagination
- providing appropriate individual support.

Training managers and line managers will also find it useful when organising the training for care and support staff.

2002 £10.80 BILD members £12.00 full price ISBN 1 904082 50 5

Autism: Early Intervention

Edited by Glenys Jones

A special supplement for the *Good Autism Practice* journal, published in 2002.

This supplement focuses mainly on the response of some local authorities in the UK to meet the needs of young children with autistic spectrum disorders and their families.

The contents of the supplement include articles on:

- Building the bridges: strategies for reaching our children
- Pre-school provision for children with autistic spectrum disorders: early intervention in Hertfordshire
- Early interventions in autism: an LEA response
- NAS EarlyBird programme: a local authority perspective
- An examination of the National Autistic Society's EarlyBird programme for parents of children with autistic spectrum disorders
- A group intervention for parents of pre-school children with autistic spectrum disorders
- Towards a model of good practice: small group early intervention for children with social communication difficulties

2002 £13.50 BILD members £15.00 full price ISBN 1 904082 66 1

To order any of these titles, please contact BILD Publications, Plymbridge Distributors, Estover Road, Plymouth, PL6 7PZ. Tel 01752 202301. Please add 10% for postage and packing for orders under £50 and 5% for orders over £50.

Good Autism Practice Journal

The first journal dedicated solely to promoting good practice with children and adults with autism and Asperger syndrome.

Good Autism Practice (GAP) will be of interest to parents and practitioners in health, education and social services, as well as people who have autistic spectrum disorders.

Published twice a year, in May and October.

For more information on *Good Autism Practice*, including subscription rates, please call BILD on 01562 723010, or email enquiries@bild.org.uk.